Counselling
for
Heart Disease

Paul Bennett

Communication and Counselling in Health Care
Series editor: Hilton Davis

Counselling
for
Heart Disease

Paul Bennett

*Principal Clinical Psychologist, Gwent Psychology Services, and
Honorary Lecturer, University of Wales College of Cardiff*

Medical advisor: Dr Alastair McDonald,
Cardiac Department, The Royal London Hospital

BPS
BOOKS
Published by the British Psychological Society

First published in 1993 by BPS Books (The British Psychological Society),
St Andrews House, 48 Princess Road East, Leicester LE1 7DR.

A catalogue record for this book is available from the British Library.

ISBN 1 85433 096 9 paperback
ISBN 1 85433 092 6 hardback

Distributed exclusively in North America by Paul H. Brookes Publishing Co., Inc.,
P.O. Box 10624, Baltimore, Maryland 21285, U.S.A.

Phototypeset by Gem Graphics, Trenance, Mawgan Porth, Cornwall
Printed in Great Britain

OTHER TITLES IN THE SERIES
Counselling Parents of Children with Chronic Illness or Disability
by Hilton Davis

To Don Sherrell

ACKNOWLEDGEMENTS

I am grateful to many people for their support and help in writing this book. In particular, thanks to Doug Carroll and John Gallacher for giving me moral support in my early ventures into research and clinical work related to cardiovascular problems. Thanks also to Hilton Davis for having the temerity to ask me to write the book in the first place, and for his constructive criticism as it has developed. Last, but not least, thanks to Helen and Tom for being there.

CONTENTS

Preface to the series   XI

Foreword by Dr Alastair McDonald   XIII

1. HEART DISEASE: CAUSES AND CONSEQUENCES   1
Risk factors for CHD   2
  Hypertension   2
  Serum cholesterol and diet   3
  Smoking   3
  Exercise   4
  Type A behaviour (TAB)   4
The impact of CHD   5
  Knowledge of risk status   5
The impact of MI   7
  The patient's experience   7
  The partner's experience   13
Implications for psychological care   14
Summary   15

2. PSYCHOLOGICAL CARE IN ACUTE SETTINGS   16
Communication-based care   16
Developing a helping relationship   18
Informational care   20
  The three-stage process   21
Emotional care   25
  Making time   30
  Enhancing control   31
Summary   33

3. A BASIC COUNSELLING APPROACH   34
Developing the helping relationship   35
A problem-solving approach to counselling   36
  Stage 1: Problem exploration and clarification   39
  Stage 2: Goal-setting   44
  Stage 3: Facilitating action   49
Summary   51

4. STRESS MANAGEMENT TRAINING   52
A model of stress   53
  Responses to stress   53

Some implications for stress management 57
Stress management and the Egan model 58
Relaxation 58
Learning relaxation skills 59
Cognitive strategies 65
Cognitive strategies and the Egan model 66
Changing self-talk 69
Cognitive challenge 72
Putting it all together 74
Rehearsal and coping 74
Reflection 76
Summary 77

5. RISK FACTOR INTERVENTION 78
Counselling smokers 78
Stage 1: Thinking about giving up 80
Stage 2: Planning to give up 81
Stage 3: Beginning to give up 82
Stage 4: 'Stop day' and beyond 85
Stage 5: Staying stopped 87
Improving fitness 88
Programme design issues 88
Generalization issues 90
Type A behaviour 92
Monitoring behaviour 94
Coping with triggers 95
Summary 100

6. PUTTING IT ALL TOGETHER 101
Organizational issues 101
Who should counsel – and why? 101
Time and space for counselling 103
Communication and adherence 103
Staff support 104
Training issues 105
Who should be counselled? 106
Referring on 107
Developing rehabilitation programmes 107
A ward-based education programme 107
A typical stress management programme 108
A minimal intervention programme 110

How effective are interventions?   110
  Psychotherapy   110
  Stress management   111
  TAB modification   112
  Exercise training   112
  Partner-based interventions   113
  Hypertension   114
Afterword   115

References   116

Appendix A: A rationale of, and preparation for, deep
  relaxation practice   119

Appendix B: Instructions for deep relaxation   121

Appendix C: An introduction to smoking cessation   124

Appendix D: Further reading   126

Index   128

LIST OF FIGURES

Figure 1: Relaxation diary recording tension ratings   62

Figure 2: Relaxation diary recording attempts to deal with tension   62

Figure 3: Example of a smoker's diary   82

Figure 4: A typical diary of Type A behaviour   95

Figure 5: Format of a typical patient education programme   108

Figure 6: A typical stress management programme   109

Preface to the Series

People who suffer chronic disease or disability are confronted by problems that are as much psychological as physical, which involve all members of their family and the wider social network. Psychosocial adaptation is important in its own right, in terms of making necessary changes in life style, altering aspirations or coping with an uncertain future. However, it may also influence the effectiveness of the diagnostic and treatment processes, and hence eventual outcomes.

As a consequence, health care, whether preventive or treatment-oriented, must encompass the psychosocial integrated with the physical, at all phases of the life cycle and at all stages of disease. The basis of this is skilled communication and counselling by all involved in providing services, professionally or voluntarily. Everyone, from the student to the experienced practitioner, can benefit from appropriate training in this area, where the social skills required are complex and uncertain.

Although there is a sizeable research literature related to counselling and communication in the area of health care, specialist texts for training purposes are scarce. The current series was, therefore, conceived as a practical resource for all who work in health services. Each book is concerned with a specific area of health care. The authors have been asked to provide detailed information, from the patient's perspective, about the problems (physical, psychological and social) faced by patients and their families. Each book examines the role of counselling and communication in the process of helping people to come to terms and deal with these problems, and presents usable frameworks as a guide to the helping process. Detailed and practical descriptions of the major qualities, abilities and skills that are required to provide the most effective help for patients are included.

The intention is to stimulate professional and voluntary helpers alike to explore their efforts at supportive communication. It is hoped that by so doing, they become sufficiently aware of patient difficulties and the processes of adaptation, and more able to facilitate positive adjustment. The aims of the series will have been met if patients and their families feel someone has listened and if they feel respected in their struggle for health. A central theme is the effort to make people feel better about themselves and able to face the future, no matter how bleak, with dignity.

Hilton Davis
Series editor

Foreword

Governments internationally are beginning to adopt long-term health strategies, undoubtedly stimulated by the initiative of the World Health Organisation, outlined in 'Health for All by the Year 2000'. Of the key areas identified, vascular disease is at the top of the list. The means of achieving health-gains in this area for the population is dependent on supportive public policies, healthier surroundings, healthy lifestyles, and high quality health services. More controversially, the specific methodology to achieve reduction in coronary heart disease and stroke is by decreasing the risk factors associated with these events. This brings into focus the confusion and disparity of views between those who adopt a policy of identifying 'high risk groups' and those who would prefer a population approach. There is also conflict, at least in emphasis, between those for whom prevention means risk factor modification, and those who prefer health promotion and the encouragement of healthy lifestyles.

Vascular disease is a physical process that has something in common with the silting up of sewers and water pipes in so far as there is an interaction between the wall of the conduit and the contents flowing past. The consequences are basically simple. Sudden occlusion (i.e. blockage) of a coronary artery causes destruction of heart muscle served by that vessel, and cardiac infarction. More gradual obstruction leads to a reduction in oxygen supply, which is less than the demand and therefore causes symptoms of angina. Age, sex, diet and cholesterol, blood pressure, smoking, exercise habit and socio-economic status are demonstrably important predictors of risk. Although emotional and psychological factors are central to risk factors such as smoking, diet and exercise, and therefore have a role in the aetiology of arterial disease, the contribution of more general personality factors remains less well defined. However, no one would deny the extent and complexity of the emotional impact of the catastrophe of heart disease on the individual, the family and on colleagues.

It is important, therefore, to address the psychological support required by victims of heart disease and their families throughout the health care process, and this book does just that. It illustrates the potential contribution to be made to those who have survived myocardial infarction, undergone cardiac surgery or other interventions. Techniques of proven benefit in risk factor modification and in the facilitation of coping techniques after illness are clearly explained. The book emphasizes how important it is for all health care professions to be aware of the extent to which they may influence the patient's response to a literally dreadful disease. The book is applicable to those working in primary care settings, including prevention, as well as hospital-based services. Good psychological care of the kind described in this book may also have more widespread benefits, in that patients convinced of their need to reform may proselytize their families and colleagues in a persuasive manner. The recently converted often wish to share their views, and this cascade of information may be a very important mechanism in spreading a change in lifestyle.

Effective counselling and communication is the key both to supporting people in trouble and persuading individuals to modify their way of life. Nurses, doctors, and all other health care professionals are becoming increasingly conscious of their responsibility to be better at reaching out, supporting, guiding, and persuading, rather than instructing and ordering. Professional groups, as well as volunteer organizations, will find this short book highly instructive and illustrative of the principles and skills of good communication and counselling.

Dr Alastair McDonald
Cardiac Department
The Royal London Hospital

1

Heart Disease
Causes and Consequences

Coronary heart disease (CHD) is at the time of writing the greatest cause of premature mortality in the Western industrialized world. It is primarily a disease of men, accounting in the United Kingdom for 40 percent of deaths in men, and 10 percent of deaths in women, aged between 45 and 64 years. In the United States, nearly one and a half million people experience myocardial infarction, of which two thirds survive.

Its most dramatic onset is in the form of acute myocardial infarction (MI). Here, an artery providing oxygen to part of the cardiac muscle (myocardium) becomes totally occluded, resulting in its death. Dependent upon the extent and site of damage, complications following MI may include altered electrical conduction of the heart, resulting in arrhythmias such as extrasystoles, tachycardia, or ventricular fibrillation. In addition, damage to the muscle may result in chronic cardiac insufficiency and heart failure. In its chronic condition, angina pectoris, episodes of insufficient blood flow to the cardiac muscle cause a number of characteristic symptoms, including chest and radiating pain and shortness of breath. These episodes may be triggered by stress, extremes of emotion (including happiness), as well as physical exertion.

About two-thirds of those who have an MI will survive and go on to achieve some degree of recovery. Approximately 16 percent of these people will suffer from angina one year later, and a further five percent will develop angina in each subsequent year. The mortality rate per year from subsequent MI is approximately five percent for older people, and under three percent for younger ones.

Some of the psychological care described in this book will address the needs of this group of survivors, particularly in helping them to come to terms with the impact of the disease, and achieving the best recovery possible. In addition, because CHD is to a large extent mediated by risk factors amenable to individual change, ways of facilitating such changes will also be discussed in the context of both preventive and rehabilitation settings.

The rest of this chapter briefly reviews the evidence linking a number of risk factors to CHD, before describing its impact on both the sufferer and their family.

Risk Factors for CHD

Three risk factors for CHD have been reliably established: hypertension, raised serum cholesterol and smoking. Two factors, Type A Behaviour (TAB) and low levels of exercise, are considered 'unproven', although it will be argued that both are important in the development of disease. In addition to these, a number of other risk factors such as age, ethnicity and social class powerfully influence risk for CHD, but are less amenable to individual change or medical treatment. Black and Asian people living in Western countries are more at risk for CHD than Caucasians, as are men, and those with manual jobs or who are unemployed. Finally, it is important to emphasize that risk factors are multiplicative. The presence of two or more risk factors confers considerably more risk than having a single risk factor.

Hypertension

There is clear evidence that raised blood pressure is related to risk for CHD and that there is a linear increase in risk as blood pressure rises. However, the greatest number of CHD–related deaths are among people with only a mildly raised diastolic pressure (90 to 104 mmHg). This is because such a large percentage of the population (up to 25 percent of adults in one study) have pressures at this level. Surprisingly perhaps, how raised blood pressure exerts its influence remains far from understood (see Beevers, 1992). It has been suggested that it is likely to lead to CHD only when serum cholesterol levels are either high, or at least at a level typical for Caucasians in Western countries. This is because high blood pressure probably leads to damage to vascular walls, which in turn leads to deposition of atheroma, particularly at arterial junctions. Other factors may also be involved, for example, people with high blood pressure have abnormal blood coagulation profiles and alterations in local tissue growth factors such as endothelin and platelet derived growth factor, which may contribute to increased atheroma.

Serum cholesterol and diet

Evidence to support the status of raised cholesterol as a risk factor for CHD is substantial. For example a four fold increase of risk for CHD between people within the lowest and highest ten percent of serum cholesterol levels has been identified. One fraction of serum cholesterol (low density lipoprotein) confers increased risk for CHD, while another (high density lipoprotein) apparently reduces risk.

More contentious, perhaps, is the relationship between *dietary* cholesterol and CHD. In a classic paper identifying risk of CHD in relation to diet, Keys (1980) reported data from seven countries that showed a positive correlation between the national average intake of saturated fat and the prevalence of heart disease-related deaths. These data have been partially replicated in a later study of European countries, although the overall relationship was not so strong and several countries were found to have very different mortality rates from that which would be predicted on the basis of the fat intake of the population. In addition, a number of longitudinal epidemiological studies have failed to find a relationship between dietary cholesterol and the incidence of CHD.

Two recent reviews in the *British Medical Journal* have critically examined research into the effects of changing cholesterol levels on risk for heart disease (Muldoon *et al.*, 1990 and Ravnskov, 1992). Both indicate the evidence is rather disappointing and that there is little to suggest that reductions in dietary intake will significantly reduce risk for heart disease. While these findings should caution against some of the strident claims made by some health-promotion programmes, they should not be taken to suggest that dietary manipulation cannot alter the course of heart disease. For example, there is strong evidence that fish oils can protect against heart disease and reduce the risk of further MI. Changes in salt intake may also reduce blood pressure.

Smoking

The first evidence to link smoking and CHD was reported in the early 1950s when nearly 188,000 healthy men were asked about their smoking habits. It was found that the risk of dying among smokers was nearly double that of non-smokers over the following four and a half years. A series of later studies have confirmed the additional risk to smokers in both men and women, and over longer periods of time. Clear evidence of a risk gradient has emerged; the more one smokes, the greater the risk for CHD (e.g. Doll *et al.*, 1980).

Other evidence supports the smoking–CHD link. Risk of death from CHD declines steadily after stopping smoking, although later studies have shown that some increased risk for CHD remains for up to 20 years after cessation. More encouragingly, the evidence suggests that the health benefits of giving up are relatively greater for younger people. In addition, among post-MI patients there is clear evidence for dramatic changes in risk status following smoking cessation (Rosenberg et al., 1990). One study found that women who continued smoking were three and a half times more at risk of re-infarction within one year than those who stopped. The relative risk dropped to two and a half times within two years of stopping, and, within three to four years, previous smoking appeared to confer little additional risk. These findings have been replicated in men.

Exercise

The first evidence that exercise may reduce the risk of CHD stemmed from studies of disease rates in sedentary and active workers. Each study revealed that people undertaking more rigorous occupational physical activity had significantly less CHD than their more sedentary colleagues. These data have now been replicated with people who engage in exercise in their leisure time. For example, it has been found that those most at risk for CHD were those who have both a sedentary job and who did not engage in vigorous exercise (Morris et al., 1980). A minimum level of exercise has to be undertaken to reduce the risk of CHD; this needs to be equal to or greater than 2,000 calories per week, the equivalent of burning off four Mars Bars!

There is increasing evidence that exercise may reduce mortality in post-MI patients; people who take part in exercise rehabilitation programmes are significantly less likely to have a further MI than those who do not (O'Connor et al., 1989). Exercise may exert its influence, at least in part, by modifying a number of risk factors for CHD progression, including weight, blood pressure, serum triglycerides and total cholesterol.

Type A Behaviour (TAB)

TAB remains one of the most controversial putative risk factors for CHD. Such behaviour comprises an excess of free-floating hostility, competitiveness, and time urgency. The archetypal Type A person is always on the go, quick to anger, and tries to fit more and more into less and less time. Early in the 1980s, TAB was acknowledged as significant a risk for CHD as hypertension, raised serum cholesterol and smoking. In particular, results from two major studies showed that Type A men and women had about double the risk for CHD than those without these characteristics (Type Bs). Risk was particularly evident amongst those whose working environment encouraged TAB.

A number of subsequent studies of post-infarction patients, however, found no relationship between TAB and re-infarction. Indeed, some found that Type Bs were more at risk. These apparently contradictory findings caused some degree of embarrassment to the Type A supporters; however, an explanation has now been given which suggests that these findings may actually support the Type A hypothesis (see Bennett and Carroll, 1990). All of these studies had a serious methodological problem; they asked patients to report their behaviour before their MI. It is possible, that while Type A behaviour contributed to the first MI, subsequent changes in behaviour (unavailable to Type Bs), either as a result of beta-blockers, self-managed change, or behavioural restrictions due to cardiac symptoms such as angina, may have protected them later.

This argument receives some support from the Recurrent Coronary Prevention Project, where changes in TAB substantially reduced the risk of recurrent MI. In addition, the only prospective study to measure behaviour as long as six months after MI found that TAB did predict re-infarction. Nevertheless, while the recent evidence does not necessarily contradict the original hypothesis, there is increasing evidence that only some aspects of TAB, particularly hostility and anger, are linked to CHD.

The Impact of CHD

As the number of people surviving major diseases has risen, so has interest in the impact of disease on their psychological and social well-being. As more people are screened to identify risk factors for CHD, with the intention that once identified these may be reduced, there is a small literature developing that examines the psychological and behavioural consequences of knowledge of risk status.

Knowledge of risk status

Screening for risk factors for heart disease is increasingly common. Most screening programmes are conducted in primary care, and comprise a brief, 20- to 30-minute, interview usually with a practice nurse.

Blood pressure and weight are measured, and dietary, exercise, and smoking habits assessed. Advice on how to reduce any risk factors is then given.

Many people who participate in such programmes are likely to have at least one risk factor for CHD. We combined data from 12 GP practices over one year and found the following prevalence rates in health checks: hypertension (newly identified), 18 percent; obesity, 42 percent; raised serum cholesterol, 27 percent; and smoking, 33 percent. This means that many people who attend health screening are likely to be given some negative health findings. They may already be aware of some factors, for example smoking and obesity. However, raised serum cholesterol and blood pressure are relatively symptom-free, and screening may be the first time that attenders are made aware of these problems.

Most people who take part in health checks find them helpful and a useful experience, and evidence is gradually accumulating to suggest that screening may facilitate some appropriate behavioural change. There is also evidence that at least some of the people made aware of their risk status are likely to find this information so threatening that they develop high levels of anxiety about their health. Unfortunately, there is good evidence that high levels of anxiety may actually prevent appropriate behaviour change, as was the case for one man who felt so frightened and overwhelmed by the knowledge of having a raised cholesterol level that he was unable to make the dietary changes that may have helped lower it. Perhaps of more concern is the fact that some people report increased anxiety about their health for some time after attending screening even where they are found *not* to be at risk. Being made aware of the potential risk to health may increase such anxieties in some people. One response to anxiety was expressed by Mr F, who illustrates the potential disruption of receiving adverse health information.

Case Study

Mr F was a 38-year-old man who attended routine screening at his GP. Until then, he considered himself quite healthy: he was not overweight, and his job, which involved some physical work, had kept him reasonably fit. It was something of a shock, therefore, when he was told that he had 'high' (7.3 mmol/litre) serum cholesterol. Mr F was given advice on how to reduce his dietary intake of saturated fat and given a list of low fat foods, with some menu suggestions. His emotional reaction to the news was not explored.

At a routine follow-up session one month later, Mr F had lost about 28 pounds, and was continuing to lose weight, despite not being previously overweight. He looked haggard, and his clothes were almost hanging off him. He said he was living almost exclusively on salads as he was unable to eat food he felt contained a significant amount of fat. His wife was experiencing considerable difficulty accommodating the various family demands in her meal preparation.

Mr F felt extremely anxious about his health in general and his cholesterol level in particular. He experienced many intrusive worries throughout the day, particularly at meal times and when he heard people discussing health matters. He said he could not help worrying he would die within the next few years unless he made radical dietary changes, as he had read that high cholesterol 'is a killer'. Without any means of judging the impact of his dietary changes on his cholesterol level, he had made a maximum effort to change.

Most people who receive adverse health information are likely to be a little anxious as a result. This is a useful reaction, as moderate and short-term increases in anxiety or concern are likely to promote appropriate behavioural change, but only when people are given help to do so. However, some people are likely to react with inappropriately high or prolonged levels of anxiety. It is important that those involved in screening are aware of the possibility of such reactions and develop a counselling style likely to promote more appropriate reactions. They should also learn to identify people who are unduly anxious before it becomes a longer-term problem.

The Impact of MI

The patient's experience

A heart attack is a physically devastating event. It is frightening, involving immediate threat to life and loss of control. It can be extremely painful. Sufferers are often surrounded by worried by-standers, rushed dramatically to hospital where they are surrounded by modern medical paraphernalia, monitored by ECG, routinely observed by nurses, and given painkilling injections that sedate and may confuse.

Although the patient is often cocooned within a Coronary Care Unit (CCU) they can usually see other patients. What they see may not be reassuring, as 20 to 30 percent of those entering a CCU are likely to die there. Equally, while many find the technology of CCUs reassuring, sophisticated technology and high levels of medical activity may reinforce the threat to life and contribute to the anxiety a patient already feels. The stress engendered by such crises may be reflected in how staff deal with other patients; it can be difficult after resuscitating (or failing to resuscitate) one patient to deal appropriately with what may seem the trivial concerns of another. Working in a CCU is a highly stressful experience, and appropriate care should be taken to meet staff as well as patient needs.

MI carries a number of meanings to the patient, most involving loss and threat; for example, loss of health, loss of status, loss of control over one's life, and the threat of future problems relating to home and work life and, ultimately, the threat of death. Such issues inevitably give rise to strong emotional reactions, which may vary from denial of the MI to acute depression and anxiety.

Denial. A surpisingly high percentage of patients (up to 20 percent in some studies) deny having had an MI. This does not mean they deny the experience of their symptoms or that they have spent time on CCU. Rather, they fail to associate their symptoms with an MI, attributing them instead to a variety of unrelated disorders or a mistaken diagnosis. This differs from suppression which involves 'trying to forget about it' or 'trying to put it to the back of one's mind'.

Short-term denial may be an appropriate and natural psychological response to overwhelming stress. Indeed, it may confer a number of advantages. Deniers report less pain and emotional disturbance in the period immediately following MI. They may return to work more quickly than those who do not deny, although not by any great margin.

However, longer-term denial may have its downside. Deniers, for example, may disregard potentially fatal symptoms, refuse appropriate medication, continue smoking, or disregard advice about appropriate exercise levels. This was certainly the case in one rehabilitation programme, which took place in a room on the sixth floor of a local hospital. All but one group member (and staff!) took the lift to get to this floor. Each week, despite advice to the contrary, one group member would arrive smiling and gasping for breath having *run* up all the flights of stairs. He was not going to let a little matter of a mistaken diagnosis of a heart attack interfere with his aerobic fitness!

Because of the psychological protection afforded by denial, some argue that it should not be challenged, and that any attempts to do so are likely to be of little value. Only where denial seems to place individuals at risk, for example, by leading to a failure to take prescribed medication, may it need to be challenged.

Anger. A second emotion likely to be experienced is that of anger. It may be turned inward as depression; it may be expressed outwardly and involve others, including friends, relatives, and staff. As heart disease is now thought, at least in part, to be preventable, so people may blame themselves for their MI. About 60 percent of people who have a heart attack attribute it to high levels of stress and overwork during the previous year, and such people may express anger both towards themselves, people who live with them, or the person who led to such overwork. The expression of anger is part of the process of dealing with the fear and other consequences of an MI; allowing patients to express their anger under controlled circumstances, such as during counselling or in the context of emotional care (see Chapter 2) may be appropriate and helpful.

Anxiety. About half the patients with MI report moderate to severe levels of anxiety while in hospital. Three to six months later this figure typically drops to one third, and to about one fifth at one year follow-up. Anxiety may present with a rise in pulse rate or blood pressure for which there is no direct medical explanation, while the patient appears overly concerned with their symptoms, bodily functions, or medication. Anxious patients may appear over dependent, demanding immediate attention and care. Many experience continuing symptoms including chest pain and weakness, which evoke high levels of anxiety. Young men, in particular, who continue to have chest pain while in hospital may experience this.

Because of the sudden and dramatic nature of the onset of disease, the real uncertainties of the future, and having perhaps too much time to think, some concerns may be exaggerated. Many patients are inclined to fantasize about permanent disablement, never being able to work again, or an inability to function as a full-fledged partner or parent. Long-term worries may come to the fore within the first day or two in CCU, as immediate worries of death and dying are added to by concerns for a future which accommodates the disease. If the person has no knowledge of the likely impact of the disease it is possible that such concerns will be unrealistic. Those who deny having an MI may be inappropriately optimistic; others inappropriately pessimistic. Some experience a short-lived anxiety when they are transferred from the apparent safety of the CCU to the general medical ward. Such anxieties are typically short lived.

Depression. Although levels of depression as high as 58 percent have been reported in CCU patients, more modest levels of between 20 to

30 percent are typical. There is, however, some evidence to suggest a small increase in the number of depressed patients up to six months after discharge. This may reflect an increasing understanding of the implications of their illness and of the disability that may result. While in hospital, the depressed person may appear to be a 'model patient', compliant, well-behaved and accepting treatment without question, when they are in reality sad, disinterested, and despondent about the future, foreseeing high risks of further infarction and disability. After discharge, they may be poor attenders to rehabilitation programmes and make few active efforts to help their progress, as people who are anxious or depressed are less likely to adhere to any rehabilitation regime than those who are less so. The following details the experiences of Mr C through the acute care stage.

Case Study

Mr C was a sales representative for a box packaging firm, admitted to the CCU late one Friday evening. During the previous weeks he had been extremely busy, and had many successful sales. On Friday he had experienced an odd chest pain during the day, but had ignored it, thinking it to be dyspepsia or some other mild ailment. However, when he got home he experienced extreme chest pain, shortness of breath, and became shocked. His wife phoned for an ambulance and Mr C was admitted as an emergency. His wife and two teenage sons followed in their car. On admission he was in tremendous pain and was highly agitated and terrified. He was given pethidine for the pain, placed on ECG, and admitted to CCU after diagnosis of MI.

During his time in CCU, Mr C felt a number of emotions, primarily fear. He felt he was close to dying, which was exacerbated by the death of a patient during his time in CCU. He remembered with terror the terrific pain he had experienced, and began monitoring himself, fearing the worst, and reporting even the smallest pain to the nursing staff.

The proximity of trained staff reassured Mr C, as he felt their specialist training and the closeness of the emergency equipment at least meant they could handle any problems he might experience. However, when he was transferred to a general medical ward three days later, he became anxious about the ability of non-specialist staff to cope with emergencies.

During the next few days Mr C began to adapt to his new situation, albeit with some difficulty. While he experienced increasing relief that he was still alive, this was mingled with worries about what the quality of that life would be. He knew his life involved high levels of stress, which he was reluctant to change as he 'thrived on it'. He thought that his physical condition might prevent him continuing his job. More immediately, Mr C was used to being in charge and in control of his life and resented being out of control. These anxieties and fears were difficult to control, and he was obviously tense and found it difficult to relax. Occasionally he would express some anger towards the nursing staff, but his fear of exacerbating his symptoms by showing his anger lead him to suppress these feelings so that most, if not all, of the staff involved in his care were unaware of how he felt.

Anxiety and negative expectations of future recovery even at the acute stage are predictive of future problems in rehabilitation. Cay *et al.* (1972) were among the first to identify two main determinants of the success of post-MI rehabilitation: the physical limitations imposed by the damaged heart muscle, and the psychological problems of accommodating to a serious illness and holding it in perspective during subsequent life. The experience of Mr T provides a good example of how anxiety which is not recognized and dealt with appropriately in acute care settings may continue to cause problems for some time after discharge.

Case Study

Mr T was 63 years old when admitted to CCU. He had had a small MI and made an uncomplicated recovery. Nevertheless, he was nervous both in the CCU and on the medical ward before discharge. He was reluctant to engage in physiotherapy, and unless directly prompted to do his exercises he remained close to his bed or seated in the dayroom. This was not seen as remarkable by the staff; no one responded to Mr T's behaviour or thought to question why he took so little exercise, and he was routinely discharged.

Some months later, following a domiciliary visit, his GP referred Mr T to the local clinical psychology department. He had become depressed and had taken early retirement. He had remained house bound since discharge and, consequently, cut off from his friends and work colleagues. Mr T had become less and less willing, or able, to do things about the house, and was increasingly bad tempered and aggressive, so that his relationship with his wife was strained. As his depression increased, his pre-occupation with cardiac symptoms worsened, and he became increasingly afraid of a further MI.

On talking to Mr T, the chain of events leading to his present state became apparent. Although his MI had been minor and had a good prognosis, he had found the episode very frightening. It had occurred following a long and tiring walk, and he also remembered previous occasions when walking or doing things about the house when he had had a 'little twinge'. During the acute recovery he had had the occasional chest pain. This combination of events and the continuing 'twinges' he continued to experience during his immediate recovery made him very anxious about 'over-exerting' himself. He became sensitized to any physical symptoms, exaggerating their significance. Mr T also took exaggerated precautions against such symptoms, avoiding even small amounts of exercise. This avoidance behaviour was reinforced by his wife, who, to calm her husband's anxieties, encouraged him to avoid even minor exertion, such as making himself the occasional cup of tea, and had taken on all the housework as well as the shopping and gardening.

Adaptation. The final stage in the process of adaptation is one of acceptance and coping with loss and changes to life. This may involve making appropriate lifestyle changes, such as stopping smoking or changing diet. For those who have severe heart disease or angina it may also involve learning to accept new limitations and accommodating to them in as positive a manner as possible. For those with less severe disease, it will involve getting back to work, but perhaps a different style of work, even if the job remains the same, where less demands are made of them.

Perhaps most of all, adaptation involves being able to live without the daily fear of recurrence. This may be difficult to achieve, and a majority of patients, even one year post-MI express concern and even anxiety about their health. One study followed up a group of MI survivors after one year and found that 34 percent of them frequently thought about heart disease; 12 percent talked about it at least several times per week; 74 percent worried about their cardiac state. If symptoms occurred, 24 percent reported a strong fear reaction. Fifty eight percent reported they were protected from physical exertion by their friends or family. It seems very difficult to forget the trauma and implications of MI.

Between 75 and 90 percent of those discharged from hospital go back to work, with white collar workers, whose jobs may be physically undemanding or who know their employers, more likely than blue collar workers to retain their job. A variety of economic factors make older patients and women less likely to return to work. Not surprisingly, people who considered work to be of central importance in their lives are likely to return to their job as early as possible.

The majority of MI patients also resume their sex life within a short time after discharge. Stern *et al.* (1976) reported that by one year post-MI, 82 percent of patients had returned to 'previous or near previous levels of sexual functioning', of which 69 percent had achieved this within 6 to 12 weeks post-MI. Somatic symptoms such as pain, breathlessness, and fatigue may well reduce the likelihood of resuming sexual activity in some people. However, fear of drastic consequences, rather than actual cardiac damage, seems to be the main obstacle in the majority of cases.

The partner's experience

It seems reasonable to direct the emphasis of both physical and psychological care towards the person who has suffered an MI. This approach, however, leads to the neglect of partners, who may also be affected by the event. While all the research has looked at the experiences of female partners of men admitted with MI, there is no reason to assume that the experiences of men whose partners – male or female – develop heart disease are any different. Indeed, as women who have an MI tend to be older, more severely ill and have a slower rehabilitation than men, partners of female MI patients may have more difficulties and require more support than those of men.

About one quarter of female partners become anxious or depressed while their male partners are in hospital, for up to one year post-MI. Women whose partners deny their infarct are particularly at risk of depression or anxiety, often feeling overwhelmed by the experience and the resulting family disequilibrium. This may be associated with high levels of strain and concern over their partner's health as a result of them not following recommended treatment regimes or engaging in risky behaviours without taking what would seem to be sensible precautions. These anxieties may be exacerbated by the women not being able to talk in any meaningful way about their partner's illness and its consequences. The story of Mrs R provides some insight into the problems such women may face.

Case Study

Mr R had a mild but definite MI about three months previously. Mrs R's mood was quite low, although she could not be described as being depressed. Nevertheless, she felt tense and stressed for much of the time. She worried about her husband, who was an active man, and felt that his admission to CCU and diagnosis of MI had been a big mistake. He attributed his symptoms at the time to severe dyspepsia, and the occasional symptoms he experienced since he felt were simply a milder form of this problem. He rarely complained of pain, although he sometimes revealed his discomfort by rubbing his chest or a slight facial grimace. Because of his unwillingness to talk about his symptoms, Mrs R had no idea how severe they were, which she found difficult to cope with.

Mr R often neglected to take medication prescribed by their GP, which was another source of anxiety for Mrs R. He also continued to smoke, despite her insistence that he at least cut down. He had made one or two desultory attempts to stop, but these had not even lasted a day. He did, however, continue to take regular exercise playing golf and occasional games of squash. When Mrs R realized he was going to play squash, she became very worried, although she hid this from Mr R because she was frightened it would result in another infarction. The whole situation was made worse by his refusal to talk about his health either with his wife or their GP.

Up to one third of female partners inhibit aggressive and sexual feelings and become overprotective of their husbands even up to one year post-MI. The quality of a relationship may also influence the social outcome of MI, although even where there is a previously poor relationship, the outcome cannot strongly be predicted. Some relationships may be further damaged by the extra strain placed; others may improve as both partners draw together to deal with these stresses.

Having a partner with CHD has some hidden costs. Many partners report an increase in household chores, although only a small percentage express dissatisfaction with this. Partners may also reduce their hours working outside the house during the early rehabilitation phase, although by one year a small number go out to work to compensate for a loss of earnings following their partner's redundancy. Older female partners of blue-collar workers suffer a greater decrease in leisure activities and in life satisfaction.

Implications for Psychological Care

As we have seen, patients in CCU and medical wards experience a range of negative emotions. These are part of the natural process of recovery from a major trauma. It is inappropriate to not feel these emotions, and if they are internalized and not expressed, they may not only add to the psychological distress associated with having had an MI, but also interfere with the rehabilitation process. In some cases they may have a profound impact on the future quality of life.

Although some people may need some form of specialist help, such as can be provided by a psychiatrist or clinical psychologist, to deal with the psychological consequences of having had an MI, many others benefit from good psychological care made available to all patients.

The main aims of psychological care should be to help individuals explore and express their feelings concerning their MI, which will facilitate active adjustment and reductions in anxiety, depression (and perhaps denial), and help them regain feelings of control over their future health and life.

Such targets can be achieved in a number of ways. Central to any approach is the development of a safe clinical environment which reassures the patient of the ward or unit's ability to cope with medical problems. In addition, patients and their relatives may benefit from good communication with staff, and from the provision of adequate formal and informal opportunities for counselling.

Gruen (1975) identified a style of approaching and interacting with those in CCU and acute wards which facilitated emotional and physical recovery that involves:

- The development of a relationship that allows the individual to talk about their concerns in a non-judgemental, accepting, atmosphere.
- Reassurance that the expression of so-called 'negative' emotions is normal, acceptable, and desirable.
- Encouragement of the patient's own coping resources.
- Acceptance of their preferred coping style; denial should not be challenged unless this interferes with medical care.
- Feedback of staff faith in the patient's ability to cope.

These and other issues are covered in the following chapters.

Summary

❑ Three primary risk factors for CHD have been identified: smoking, hypertension and raised serum cholesterol.

❑ The available evidence suggests two other factors may also be strongly implicated in the development of disease: low levels of exercise and TAB. All of these may be modified by behavioural change, suggesting that such changes may either prevent disease or disease progression following infarction.

❑ A number of adverse psychological consequences to MI have also been identified, in particular: depression, anxiety, and anger, each of which may adversely affect rehabilitation. The consequences of denial are more complex, but may also compromise rehabilitation.

❑ Not only is the impact of MI on the patient potentially severe, but partners and families may also experience adverse consequences.

❑ Good psychological care should be available to all patients.

2

Psychological Care in Acute Settings

Good psychological care may positively affect the individual's psychological and physical state whilst in hospital and perhaps more importantly, may profoundly alter future prognosis and longer term rehabilitation. Some patients in CCUs, acute medical wards, or undergoing Coronary Artery Bypass Graft (CABG) operations, may benefit from specialist treatment for emotional problems. Their distress may be clear, and their need for some form of psychological help obvious. Their needs, however, should not distract from those of the majority. They may not experience the same extremes of emotional distress, but may also benefit from help in reducing psychological stress and promoting healthy psychological recovery following the acute stage of their illness.

A major source of reassurance to both patients and their relatives is the knowledge that they are in a safe clinical environment which can cope with medical problems. Assuming this to be the case, a number of other factors relating to the psychological care of the patient become salient. Two key aspects involve informational and emotional care. A further dimension, that of optimizing individuals' perceptions of control over their environment and rehabilitation is also important. The rest of this chapter focuses on skills pertinent to each of these aspects of care. The skills described under each heading are not only pertinent to that aspect of care; rather, they provide stepping stones to an integrated model of patient care in which any of the skills described can be used whenever necessary.

Communication-based Care

Talking to patients and their relatives is often assumed to be straightforward, barely worth a thought, and assumed to occur effectively with little or no training. Nothing could be further from the truth. One of the most frequently-cited causes of patient dissatisfaction with health care is poor staff–patient communication. The basics of good communication underpin all later discussions of differing communication issues, and some will be discussed in more detail as the book progresses.

Effective communication-based care requires both appropriate organizational structures and personal qualities of those involved in its provision.

Organizational issues include:

- communication-based care being perceived as central to good patient care;
- being proactive in the delivery of communication-based care;
- allowing time and privacy for effective care.

Personal skills common to all communication-based care include establishing a helping relationship through, among other ways:

- showing warmth and friendliness;
- communicating understanding and empathy;
- verbal and non-verbal listening skills.

To be effective, informational and emotional care should be seen as central to patient care. In addition, it is important that all those involved with patients and relatives actively engage in effective communication. The quality of such care is only as good as its weakest link. It is also important to co-ordinate this type of care much as any other patient-oriented activity. It should not be assumed to happen by default. Neither can it be conducted appropriately during other routine duties. At a minimum, these will interfere with the smooth flow of conversation and may well deter patients from asking questions, as they may not wish to hold up the carer from other, obviously pressing, tasks. Attention should also be paid to privacy, carrying out such types of care in a separate room.

Because it is important that *all* those involved in patient care develop and use good communication skills, the following examples of their use involve all members of the professions involved in the care of patients with heart disease. To further denote the multi-disciplinary nature of the communication skills discussed, the text will refer to anyone involved in patient care as a 'carer' and avoid note of their discipline or background.

Developing a Helping Relationship

The key to all communication-based care is the development of a good relationship between the carer and patient and any other people who are involved with them. The importance of this relationship may vary according to the depth and length of care being provided. Nevertheless, the effectiveness of *any* helping relationship will be governed, to a large extent, by the ability of the carer to achieve a good relationship. Without a degree of trust and liking, people will be reluctant to engage in any dialogue and unwilling to talk about issues that are troubling them.

Being friendly and warm can be a useful initial help in developing a relationship. People are more likely to respond positively to someone who smiles and greets them cheerfully than to a morose and dour person. However, care should be taken not to extend a false bonhomie:

Patient: *I know I drink too much, and smoke too much too. But you know, I've tried to cut down and it's really hard.*

Nurse: *Yes I know. But most smokers find it difficult to stop – and that goes for many drinkers too. Don't feel so bad about it.*

Here, the nurse's comments, while trying to be sympathetic and nice are veering towards the sycophantic and positively unhelpful. The goal of communication in this context is not necessarily to provide a sympathetic ear that serves to maintain or even encourage the *status quo*. It may be necessary, at times, to challenge attitudes or beliefs particularly in more goal-oriented counselling sessions (see page 44).

Another important way in which a helping relationship can be achieved is through developing empathy. This means trying to pick up what the person is saying and showing, and to identify how they are feeling; that is to see the story from their perspective. Echoing this understanding helps engage the person, makes them feel safe, and encourages them to explore any issues further. One simple way in which empathy can be communicated is by occasionally reflecting back, perhaps with some elaboration, what the patient has told you they are experiencing.

Patient: *Sometimes, at the end of the day I feel that I've put so much energy into doing some work, with very little to show for it. Yet I'm far more tired than I ever was before my heart attack.*

Doctor: *It sounds like you feel really frustrated that you can't do as much in the day as you used to . . .*

Patient: *Yes, I do. And then I get worried that my boss may give me the sack . . . and that winds me up even more.*

Merely paraphrasing back what a person has told you may feel like a mechanistic approach to counselling. Indeed, it can become a sterile technique. However, if used appropriately, for example in reflecting back on part of a dialogue, it can show a person the listener's under-standing of the person's situation and their feelings. As in the above example, it may be a powerful factor in helping them explore their problems or feelings, and may promote exploration of a problem more than a more direct question. Finally, it can provide important feedback to the carer as to whether they are truly understanding. If the person frequently denies the reality of their experiences reflected back to them ('No, that's not how it feels . . .') this may be a signal that he or she is not gaining sufficient empathy.

Empathy is *not* communicated through phrases such as, 'I know what you're going through', or, 'I understand'. The carer may have some appreciation of the person's experience. However, most people cannot fully understand. Repetition of such trite phrases may prove alienating: 'No! You *don't* understand. How could you?'. (Further ways of developing and expressing empathy are described in Chapter 3.)

Non-verbal behaviour can also affect the quality of a relationship. During normal conversation, it is often possible to see that someone has lost interest in what is being said. They may move slightly away from the speaker, or begin to look away more frequently. To the sensitive speaker, these non-verbal cues act as signals to end the con-versation and move on. Similarly, it is possible to use non-verbal behaviour to show interest and care. Without such cues, a person may be unwilling to explore personal issues or problems. Non-verbal behaviour acts as a signal of intent, and may facilitate or interfere with the communication process. Non-verbal behaviour can be used to enhance the helping relationship by:

➤ facing the person squarely;
➤ adopting an open posture;
➤ leaning slightly forwards;
➤ maintaining good eye contact;
➤ trying to be relaxed.

The most obvious thing when looking at two people in conversation is their position relative to each other. Interest in what is being said is shown by standing close and looking at the person speaking. In effec-tive communication-based care, the carer needs to be in a posture of involvement, oriented towards the person or at right angles to them. This allows each person to see the other fully and to achieve and break eye contact, but does not lead to direct face-to-face contact, which some people find confrontational.

Crossed arms and legs can be a signal of a closed conversation, and imply low involvement. A more open posture carries a message that the carer is actively engaged and interested in what a person has to say. Equally, leaning a little forward indicates interest, while leaning back, easy to do if a conversation is conducted in easy chairs, may imply boredom or a failure to engage.

Eye contact is also an important signal during normal conversation implying interest and engagement. If a carer breaks or avoids contact this may imply a lack of interest or that they wish to speak. Maintaining steady eye contact, albeit with occasional looks away to avoid staring or during changes of speaker, is an important facilitating factor.

Finally, it is important to be relaxed. You may have other things to do, or may be worried about what to do in the session, but this should not be transmitted through fidgety or anxious behaviour, which will simply confuse, or make the person anxious, and lessen the value of the session.

Informational Care

Patients being admitted to hospital for relatively routine and planned procedures such as CABG may well have many questions they wish to ask, and issues they wish to discuss. Patients in CCUs, and their relatives, are likely to be even more anxious and bewildered by events. The process of admission is usually dramatic, and there is little time to provide full explanations of exactly what is happening, let alone what is likely to happen, to worried relatives or the patient. Nevertheless, even at this early stage many people are brimming with questions about both the short-term as well as the long-term implications of MI. 'Will he be all right?', 'Is he going to die?', 'Will he be able to go back to work?', 'How long will he be in hospital for?' All these are important questions for both the patient and their relatives. Some may be simple to answer. Others, for example those relating to future prognosis, may be more difficult. If information is given carefully and sensitively, it may positively aid psychological adjustment and promote active engagement in the rehabilitation process. Inappropriate communication may fail to relieve confusion and fear, or may even add to them.

In hospital there is typically a basic inequality of information: doctors usually know the most information about a patient's condition and likely prognosis, nurses and other care providers may know somewhat less, although in specialized areas, such as coronary care, they may know as much as some doctors. At the bottom of the hierarchy is the patient, who generally knows very little about their case!

Although they may want appropriate information, many patients feel unable to seek it. They may lack the assertive skills required, or not want to 'bother' obviously busy staff. They may also be so debilitated by their condition that they have no energy to invest in seeking information. Yet without it, they may develop inappropriate anxieties or be unaware of their potential for recovery. Consequently, they will not be able to fully engage in the recovery process.

For these reasons, information should not be given only when patients or their relatives make particular efforts to seek it. Good informational care should be proactive: it should be assumed that most people want information, and at a level appropriate to their knowledge and ability to understand and cope with it. However, a small percentage of people cope best by avoiding information. They do not want to be confronted with information on their condition. Forcing unwanted information on them may actually increase their anxiety and concerns. For example, most people will find it extremely helpful to be told what to expect before and after CABG surgery. A minority of people, however, find this information worrying, even distressing; they would rather not know. For this reason it is important to check how much patients know, and what they *want* to know, before providing information.

The three-stage process

Nichols (1984) has identified a three-stage process to informational care:

- Initial check of the person's present level of knowledge.
- Information exchange.
- Accuracy check: making sure any new information has been remembered and understood.

Initial check. Before giving information it is important to find out what the person already knows and what they want to know. This may avoid unnecessary reiteration and providing contradictory information. It also gives some clues about the level at which information should be pitched.

It is important that questions asked by the carer are 'open' questions, which invite full answers and not 'closed' ones which allow 'yes' and 'no' answers. It should not be assumed that the person remembers information given previously. Anxiety, drugs which control pain, and a host of other factors may mean that information has been forgotten. Because people may feel embarrassed or unwilling to seek information about something both they and the carer know they have already been told, it may be best to avoid questions which hark back to previous information exchanges, for example: 'Can you remember what Sister James told you about your condition when you discussed it yesterday?' This sounds a bit like a test, with marks given for accuracy! It is also a closed question, inviting a minimal answer. Much better would be a question such as:

Nurse: *I know you spoke to Sister James about your condition yesterday, but I don't know exactly what she told you. Could you tell me what you talked about? Or if you have thought of any questions about what you discussed, perhaps I could answer them now.*

This is much more inviting and will put the person at ease, so they will be more likely to ask questions about concerns they have and to benefit from any information exchange.

This stage can also be used to find out whether the person wants more information, or whether they have sufficient for that time. If they do not want more at this time, it should not be assumed that they will not wish information in the future, and further checks will still need to be made.

Information exchange. Once it has been established what a person knows or wishes to know, appropriate information can be given. This sounds simple, but again some thought has to be given as to how information is given to make it both understandable and memorable.

The language used has to be appropriate to the person to whom the information is being given. Note must be taken of the level of understanding and language used by the person and the level of technicality altered accordingly. For example, it is clearly inappropriate to discuss a 'myocardial infarction' or 'transient ischaemia' with a person who has little understanding of how the heart works. Similarly, to tell a patient they have been prescribed beta-blockers or diuretics may confer absolutely no information to them whatsoever. Here are a few rules of thumb that will help effective information exchange:

➤ Do not overload people with information.
➤ Information should be expressed clearly in short and simple sentences.
➤ The language used should mirror that of the person.
➤ Diagrams and notes may help explanations and aid memory.
➤ Information should be provided coherently, issue by issue, not as a jumble of related and unrelated bits of information.
➤ Repetition increases memory. To misquote a famous dictum: 'Tell 'em what you're going to tell 'em, tell 'em, and tell 'em what you've told 'em'.

Some of these points are exemplified by the following conversation between a doctor in CCU and Mr T:

Doctor: *We talked yesterday about your heart attack and what is likely to happen to you over the next few days in hospital. I know your wife came to see you yesterday evening, and I was sorry not to have a chance to speak to her. Did she have any questions she wants answering, or have you thought of any more questions since we last spoke?*

Mr T: *Yes. She was a bit concerned about my medicine. As you know I'm still getting some pain and she thought I may not be getting the right tablets. She was also a bit worried that I'm still attached to the heart monitor. Oh yes, and I've been worrying about my son. He's getting married soon and I'm a bit worried about whether I'll be able to get to the wedding. What do you think?*

Doctor: *Hmmm . . . That's quite a bit to talk about! OK, let's do it in stages. First, I can understand you're worried about the pains you're getting. I'll try and explain why you're still getting them, and hopefully show you that they're not related to your tablets. Then we can discuss your tablets and why you're still on a monitor if you still want to. That may take a fair amount of time, so can I suggest we talk about your son's wedding later on today? If you or your wife wish we can talk about any of these things at visiting time as well.*

Note how the doctor clearly delineated what he would explain first, second, and so on. Importantly, she agreed first to explain why Mr T was still getting some chest pains. If she had not done so, Mr T's anxiety about the pain may have interfered with his concentrating on, and remembering, any other information he was given. Finally, to avoid information overload she broke the information exchange into two sessions.

Accuracy check. Patients and relatives may nod their heads in the right places and appear to have understood everything they are told.

However, this may not be the case, and should never be assumed. It can be checked by, for example, asking patients to repeat information and assess its accuracy. Where errors are made, the opportunity can be taken to correct or clarify issues which may not have been understood. This needs to be done implicitly and with tact; care should be taken that this stage is not seen by the person as a 'test' or felt to be patronizing.

Mr F was admitted to CCU and had been there for one day. A nurse co-ordinating his information care had the following dialogue with him:

Nurse: *Well, you've been with us for a day now, and quite a lot has happened to you. It must have been a confusing and anxious time for you.*

Mr F: *You can say that again! It's pretty frightening being here. What's likely to happen to me?*

Nurse: *That's a big question! Would you like to know about what's likely to happen to you while you're in coronary care, or are there other things you would like to know about?*

Mr F: *Let's talk about what to expect here first.*

Nurse: *OK. Can you just remind me what you were told yesterday? Perhaps I could fill in some of the gaps or make it clearer than we may have done then.*

Mr F: *Well, to be quite honest I can't remember very much of what I was told yesterday. It's all been pretty confusing. My memory's not that good at the best of times, let alone now.*

Nurse: *That's understandable. Most people feel that way for the first few days. Let me tell you about the things around your bed. This is the heart monitor. It's attached to these wires on your chest and takes readings of the activity of your heart, allowing us to monitor your progress. If you look, there is a peak every time your heart beats, followed by a little wavy line before the next. This shows the electrical activity of the heart as it beats and then rests in between beats.*

Mr F: *Does this mean I may have another heart attack?*

Nurse: *That's unlikely given the state of your heart, although it's possible. Most people with a heart attack similar to yours go on to make a full recovery. The good thing about being attached to the monitor is that it allows us to see things developing, so we can give you treatment to prevent them becoming real problems.*

Mr F: *That's a relief!*

The nurse continues to tell Mr F about the unit, its routine, and so on. She is now coming to the end of giving information, and needs to check whether Mr F would like any further information, and to ensure that he has understood what she has said:

Nurse: *Well! I think that's about all that's worth saying at the moment. Is there anything else you would like to know about?*

Mr F: *Not that I can think of right now.*

Nurse: *Well you can always ask me another time. I expect your wife is going to ask you about some of the things I've told you when she visits. Let's check that I've been clear and not given you too much to take in at once. Imagine that I'm your wife . . .*

Mr F: *Chance would be a fine thing!*

Nurse (laughs): *Steady on! Why don't you explain to me the things we've talked about as you will later on, just to make sure I haven't confused you or been unclear.*

Even this short dialogue raises a number of issues. First, it illustrates the fact that informational care is conducted in parallel with other psychological care. In this case, Mr F expressed anxiety about his condition, which may, or may not, have been allayed by the information he was given. Further exploration of these worries may have been beneficial, and an alert carer may have moved to these after the informational care phase, or even allowed them to take priority and tackled these issues instead of simply providing more information.

Second, while the nurse was reassuring whenever possible, she did not pull back from the truth. She admitted the possibility of a further MI, although providing appropriate information and reassurance of the low risk at the same time. This may have been a good time to explore some of Mr F's anxieties and concerns, particularly in relation to his future prognosis. Finally, although the context was serious and the dialogue was conducted in a professional manner, some humour was injected into the situation. Matters may be serious, but they do not necessarily have to be dealt with in a solemn manner. In this case the humour was quite appropriate as it matched – indeed, responded to – the patient's style and approach to the situation.

Emotional Care

Emotional care involves enabling people to talk about their feelings and emotions. Most of us 'feel better for a little weep' when things get us down. Following the expression of negative emotions there is often a resurgence of more positive feelings, and this is also true for individuals experiencing emotional distress.

Negative emotions such as fear, anxiety or anger form part of the psychological response to serious illness, in particular one with such potentially overwhelming consequences as an MI. Getting in touch with and expressing these feelings is part of the healing process. Keeping these feelings in may inhibit the process of recovery. For example, fears may become enlarged and more debilitating. Depressive thoughts may become more real if they are internalized, brooded upon, and not expressed. The experience of many patients is that talking to someone about their fears and worries allows them not to think about them at other times. It stops them ruminating and, paradoxically, helps them to be more positive in their outlook.

Those who admit to, or talk about, their worries and fears should not be labelled as 'neurotic' or 'difficult'. Equally, it must not be assumed that those who openly express such emotions are the only people who experience distress, or would benefit from talking about their fears and concerns. Many people feel inhibited in expressing emotions, particularly in settings such as hospitals that traditionally do not facilitate their expression. Full patient care should therefore permit, or even encourage, the expression of such emotions. It should not simply be targeted at those who evidence high levels of psychological distress, but be central to the care of all patients.

This approach is in some conflict with the more traditional approach to emotional care which is implemented only when a person is in emotional pain, and has as its primary goal the direct amelioration of distress, often by trying to find something which feels helpful. This approach frequently results in the immediate inhibition, but not reduction, of distress rather than helping in its resolution.

Emotional support involves offering time, and using that time to absorb what people say, to understand, empathize, and gently assist them in confronting and expressing their feelings. It does not mean taking over a person's problems and trying to solve them, or giving them treatment to reduce stress. There are a number of key elements to emotional care. These include:

- Making the situation safe.
- Giving permission for the expression of emotion.
- Sharing emotional responses.

Making the situation safe. The foundation of emotional care is for a person to feel safe; that is, they feel they will not be judged, embarrassed, or devalued if they express worries, weakness, or anxieties. This involves not challenging or devaluing their experience, but accepting their emotions and concerns without judging or trying to allay them. The focus of the communication should be on the individual's experience, not on the professional's (in the case below, an occupational therapist) attempts to alleviate or solve problems, at least before these are fully explored:

Mr L: *I'm really worried that I won't be able to go back to my old job. I'll have to take a pay cut or go on the dole.*

OT: *Come on . . . It'll probably be all right. You'll get back. Now come on! Don't worry about that.*

Here, the OT has tried, admittedly in a rather clumsy way, to reassure Mr L that his worries are unfounded. However, he has done this from a position of total ignorance of his situation. It is an immediate response, which essentially rejects Mr L's feelings, and makes him most unlikely to express other concerns that he may have, or distress he may be feeling. A response which would be more likely to facilitate Mr L's expression of emotional distress would be more accepting of the reality of his distress:

OT: *That sounds like a big issue for you. Why don't you think you'll be able to get back to work?*

And, later.

OT: *How do you feel about this – anxious, angry?*

Note that much of the feedback of safety is based on the expression of empathy, rather than sympathy.

Permission to express emotion. Our culture does not encourage the expression of emotional upset. Even at times of crisis, people may apologize for the 'unseemly' expression of feelings, such as crying or feeling angry. This ethos is carried through to hospitals. It is ironic that in most hospitals, where extremes of sadness and joy are frequently experienced, so little regard is paid to dealing with them. The atmosphere of a hospital typically constrains the expression of both types of emotion.

Emotional care demands just the opposite, and because it is counter to the norms of society at large and typical hospital care in particular, clear permission for the expression of emotions may be necessary. This is not to say that emotional care demands a clear statement of permission ('OK, Mr Jones, it's emotional care time. Please feel free to pour your heart out to me ...!'). Instead, this type of permission is more subtle and dependent on reactions to information given by patients in the course of wider conversations.

Giving permission to express emotions, and particularly negative emotions, involves a number of skills, including:

• Gentle questioning.
• Showing empathy.
• Allowing time for the expression of emotion.
• Not interfering.
• Not trying to allay or inhibit distress.

The beginnings of permission may be direct or indirect. If a patient shows evident signs of distress, it may be sufficient to show you have noticed this and have time to talk about any concerns they may have. A direct approach may be particularly useful if the patient and carer have already begun to establish a helping relationship. This could start with an empathic statement, if necessary followed by a gentle, but more direct question:

Doctor (gently): *Hello, Mr J. I've noticed you a couple of times today looking sad ... Is anything troubling you?*

Sometimes, hidden concerns or distress may become apparent in the course of other conversations, and the carer may move the conversation to an exploration of this upset. In the earlier case of Mr F (page 24), who expressed some anxiety about his condition and appeared somewhat alarmed when the reasons for being on a monitor were described to him, this may be taken as a sign to complete the information exchange before exploring some of his concerns. Again, this may start with an empathic statement, or a direct question:

Doctor: *You seemed quite alarmed when we were talking earlier about being in Coronary Care ...* or,

Doctor: *Is anything in particular worrying you about your condition or treatment?*

The expression of concerns or emotion is not always easy. Accordingly, it is important that emotional care is not rushed, and that time is given to ensuring people have time to explore and express their feelings. This may mean that a conversation is punctuated with pauses. There is often the temptation to fill these pauses and to maintain the flow of dialogue. In fact, these may be the most important part of the whole process. The skill of the carer is often simply to sit quietly and to share the feelings of the person, letting them express them in their own time. Hasty interruptions or questions by the carer will simply prevent, or at least interfere with, the expression of emotion.

It is also important that non-verbal behaviour is in keeping with the verbal content of any dialogue. The carer should be still and quiet, maintaining occasional eye contact. Gentle physical contact, for example, a hand placed gently on the person's arm, may provide all the empathy needed at times of strong emotion. Some of these points are illustrated in the case of Mr W:

Mr W: *This is crazy. Here I am, a young man, and I know the Doc says I've only had a minor heart attack. But I just can't help feeling that this is it. I'm condemned to a life with no future! I won't be able to play football again, my work's going to go downhill! Jeez, I could die at any time!*

Nurse: *Sits quietly and rests his hand on Mr W's arm.*

Mr W: *I'm sorry. I didn't mean to go on like that. It's just that these feelings come over me – and I can't hold them in.*

Nurse (quietly, to match Mr W's mood): *That's OK. You were saying you felt condemned to a life with no future . . .*

Mr W: *Yes! Well, and no. Sometimes I feel like that. The feeling just pops up. Something I hear or think, and I just can't shake it. Do you know what I mean?*

Nurse: *I think so. It must make you feel very anxious . . .*

In this dialogue, the nurse listens and accepts, almost without comment, what Mr W tells him. He does not try to reassure or contradict. Instead he accepts and empathizes with his feelings. He shows some empathy by simply touching his arm, as if to say 'I am here and listening'. He accepts his emotions, and gently encourages him to express his upset by reflecting back his feelings in an attempt to encourage him to explore them further.

Sharing emotional responses. So far, the role of the carer in emotional care has been primarily described as that of a caring, but relatively neutral, facilitator of emotional expression. An understanding of the person's perspective is given through reflecting back their own statements and concerns.

I have already warned against the use of comments such as 'I understand', or, 'I know what you're going through'. Sometimes, however, it can be useful to show your own feelings or emotional response to a person's situation, for example, by being quiet, smiling or showing sadness. While too much involvement may disrupt a helping relationship – it is after all a professional relationship between patient and health care provider – the occasional expression of emotion in response to a person's story, be it sadness, anger or even joy, may help build a genuine trusting relationship, which is the key to full emotional care.

Such expression should not take the form of claiming an understanding of the person's feelings or situation. Rather it should be a genuine reflection of your own response to what you have been told: Physiotherapist: *'That must be very difficult to cope with. I feel very sad after hearing about* ... Of course, not everything is sad, and it is sometimes rather more pleasant to acknowledge your pleasure about a good thing which has happened: Doctor: *'That's great! I'm really happy for you'.* The most important thing about this aspect of emotional care is that the response is your own genuine one. If you feel powerfully moved, say so.

Making time

Just as in providing informational care, time has to be allocated to the provision of emotional care. It cannot be conducted at the same time as other patient-oriented tasks, which will distract from the process and make emotional care of little or no benefit. How much time should be spent with each person should be determined by both the professional time available and the needs of the individual. Some people cope well with any problems and need a minimum of emotional care. They will need little more than occasional brief meetings to enquire, at a personal level, how they are getting on and, in doing so, reassuring them of your ongoing concern.

On the other hand, a sizeable proportion of seriously ill people are likely to be experiencing great emotional upheaval. In such cases, early contact with frequent meetings are the ideal; say, once a day for a brief period, with longer sessions less frequently. Each session should be uninterrupted wherever possible. To make the most of these sessions, people should be given some idea of the time available to them, so they can use it to its full.

A session in which emotional care is given can be demanding to both person and carer. Because of this, it is important to ensure that any session does not finish at a time of great emotional distress. If someone has shown distress and upset during a session, care must be taken to lighten the mood before the session ends:

Nurse: *We must finish in a few minutes, I'm afraid. Perhaps we need to spend the last few minutes of the session looking back at what we've discussed, and seeing how you feel about them.*

Mr G: *Yeah. I'm sorry to have gone on like that . . .*

Nurse: *There's no need to apologize. It's important that you let these feelings out.*

Mr G: *Yeah. I guess so. It was pretty hard though.*

Nurse: *It felt that way at times . . . How are you feeling now? You'll be going back to the main ward in a minute. Will you be all right?*

Mr G: *I think so . . . If it's all right with you, I'll just spend a few minutes on my own to get my thoughts in order.*

Nurse: *That's a good idea. Take as long as you want. If you would like, we can have another session in a couple of days' time. In the meantime, if you need to talk anything through let me know and I'll try to make some time. OK?*

Mr G: *Fine. Thanks a lot.*

Enhancing control

An important factor in recovery from any major illness is a belief in one's ability to do something positive, either in terms of preventing a recurrence or in achieving a good recovery. Without this belief, patients are likely to become passive recipients of care and disengage from the rehabilitation process. This disengagement may not be immediately apparent. Patients may participate in whatever rehabilitation activities are required of them. However, they may do so with little enthusiasm, and, more worryingly, take little or no initiative in them. This may have no immediate consequences. However, away from the encouragement of the hospital setting, they may not be motivated to make the best of their chances, may become dependent on others, and make a less than optimal recovery.

A central goal of rehabilitation, therefore, is to encourage active engagement in recovery and to enhance patients' perceptions of control and responsibility for their future well-being. From the very start of the rehabilitation process, patients should be involved in, and given some responsibility for, their care. This will prevent them adopting a stance of passive acceptance of their treatment, and from the start will show the need for them to become actively involved. Such responsibility may be small, certainly in the early stages of care, but should be obvious and shown to be important. Initially, this may mean asking patients to engage in some part of their required programme in their own time. For example, they may be asked to engage in routine passive exercises once each hour. Of course, it will be a responsibility of the ward staff to ensure these are actually conducted. However, if they forget, patients may be gently reminded to do them ('How are the exercises going?') rather than told ('Don't forget to do your exercises'), or more forcibly reminded ('Have you done your exercises yet?'). The differences between these approaches may appear small and irrelevant. However, the first implicitly assumes the patient will accept, or has accepted, responsibility for this aspect of their care. The latter implicitly suggests that the professionals still have control. If each type of message is sustained over the period of hospitalization, the degree of responsibility a patient takes for their rehabilitation may be very different.

As patients recover, they can be involved in making decisions about many aspects of their treatment. This is not to say they should be asked to make decisions about aspects of their care about which they have no knowledge. This could have calamitous medical consequences! However, there are many aspects of care, about which, with some information, they may make some decisions. For example, rather than having a standard routine of walking a set amount each day, individuals can be involved in deciding how much exercise they feel they can handle. Their decisions may then be negotiated, if necessary, with the care provider. Critical to such negotiation is that the carer asks the patient about *their* choice of action, and appropriate information to inform any decisions is given:

Physiotherapist: *We need to start thinking about how much you should exercise over the next couple of days. How much do you feel up to doing?*

Mr Q: *I haven't really thought about that . . . A ten-mile jog? (laughs) No, seriously, I suppose I could walk two or three times up and down the corridor outside the ward.*

Physiotherapist: *Hmm . . . I'm glad to see you're so keen, but that sounds a little enthusiastic. Most people just walk up and down the corridor once, but do this three or four times a day.*

Mr Q: *OK. I'll stick to that for today. But tomorrow, I hope I can do rather more.*

Physiotherapist: *Fine. But let's see how you go today before we make a decision.*

This type of approach has a number of advantages: it involves the patient in decision-making, and nurtures responsibility and confidence in decisions they will have to make on their own when discharged. It also allows staff to identify (and pre-empt) the possibility of future problems if the patient is either unduly pessimistic or optimistic about how much they should be doing.

Summary

❑ Three approaches to care in acute settings have been identified. A basic requirement of all these types of care is the development of a *helping relationship* with the patient, which can be achieved, in part, through:

– a warm and friendly approach;
– showing empathy with the patient;
– non-verbal behaviour which shows interest in what is being said.

❑ Informational care comprises three phases:

– Initial check: involves finding out what the patient already knows and what they wish to know.
– Information exchange: patients should not be overloaded with information, and language used should be appropriate. Diagrams and notes may help explanations and aid memory.
– Accuracy check: care should be taken to ensure people have understood what they have been told. They can be asked (subtly!) to repeat information, with corrections made where necessary.

❑ Emotional care involves allowing the expression of emotional distress as a way of helping patients come to terms with their illness. As well as depending heavily on empathy, at least three other skills will enable this type of care:

– making the situation safe;
– giving permission for the expression of emotion, through gentle questioning, not interfering with the expression of emotion, allowing time for the expression of emotion;
– sharing emotional responses.

❑ Enhancing control and personal responsibility is an important factor in rehabilitation. This can best be achieved by giving patients some negotiated responsibility for their care. Wherever possible, patients should be enabled to make decisions about their treatment.

3

A Basic
Counselling Approach

To many people, counselling is synonymous with advice-giving ('If I were you, I would . . .', 'What I think you should do is . . .'). However, nothing could be further from the truth. The essence of counselling is to form a helping relationship which actively encourages the person being counselled to identify *their own* solutions to particular problems. Counselling can be as brief as one conversation or it may extend over a period of time. Counselling methods can be used in a variety of settings, and with problems as varied as helping someone to stop smoking or to cope with emotional distress.

The term counsellor has a number of connotations. It may indicate that a person has had a formal training in counselling techniques or provides a specialist counselling service. The goal of this chapter is to give the reader an understanding of some of the basic techniques used in counselling and to encourage the use of these methods in everyday care. It is not intended to make the reader 'a counsellor'. Nor is it intended that the use of these techniques should be restricted to a few specialist workers. Rather, it is hoped that many of the people involved in patient care, either in preventive or acute settings, will be able to use these skills when, and where, necessary. Accordingly, the text will refer to anyone engaged in the process of counselling as a 'helper'. This seems most appropriate, as the ultimate goal of counselling is to help the individual determine their own solutions to the problems they face. The role of the person with whom they interact is simply to facilitate this process.

Gerald Egan's book, *The Skilled Helper* (Egan, 1990), is a synthesis of a number of therapeutic approaches, and provides a good framework upon which to build the helping process. It has two fundamental tenets. Firstly it is person-centred; the helper does not act as an expert who can solve the person's problems, or even provide advice about how they should set about doing so. Instead, the helper's role is to facilitate the individual's *own* resources both to identify problems and arrive at strategies of how to solve them. The second tenet is that the counselling process is problem-oriented: the goal of counselling is to identify problems in the here and now, and to develop strategies to resolve them. It is, therefore, applicable to a wide variety of problems and issues, and in both primary care and acute care settings.

Some aspects of relationship building were described in Chapter 2. Because of the fundamental importance of these, some further related issues will be discussed, before looking in some detail about how these and other skills may be used within the counselling framework as developed by Egan.

Developing the Helping Relationship

Carl Rogers and others have emphasized three fundamental characteristics of good helpers, who must:

* respect their patients;
* empathize with their patients;
* be genuine in their counselling relationships.

Respect implies that the helper cares about a person's welfare, can see them as a unique human being, not simply a 'case', and perceives them as capable of determining their own fate. Respect can be shown by: attending and listening actively to what the person says; suspending critical judgement; communicating empathy; helping them to identify and cultivate their own resources; and by providing encouragement and support throughout the counselling process.

Genuineness means being natural and open in your counselling relationship with people. This can be shown by not over-emphasizing the professional role, being spontaneous but not uncontrolled or haphazard, and being willing to share your own feelings and experience if this may be helpful.

Empathy is not simply acknowledging the other person's experience. It involves gaining an understanding, *from their perspective*, of what has happened to them, and the emotional impact of this.

Occasionally, there may be apparent conflicts between some of these attributes. Some helpers may find it difficult, for example, to counsel smokers or people who are obese, feeling it is the person's own stupidity or lack of control which has resulted in their problems. Being genuine would mean that they express some of these feelings, which could inhibit or even prevent the development of a helping relationship. For this reason if carers feel very strongly about such matters, it may be inappropriate for them to counsel the people towards whom they feel this way. However, it may be possible to resolve this apparent conflict by being respectful of the person as someone with many facets and characteristics, while being genuine in not condoning their behaviour.

Another attribute that will enhance a helping relationship is the perceived trustworthiness of the helper. This may be encouraged by:

- being sensitive to the person's needs and feelings;
- demonstrating genuineness and sincerity;
- being realistic, but optimistic, about people's abilities to get to grips with the problems they face;
- maintaining confidentiality;
- making a contract and keeping any agreements made.

Confidentiality is a particularly fraught topic in hospitals, particularly for nursing and other so-called paramedical staff. Doctors have always been bound by the Hippocratic oath, which states that what they are told by a patient is confidential and must not be disclosed. Issues of confidentiality among the so-called paramedical staff have been, and in some cases remain, less clear. However, the codes of practice for an increasing number of professions, such as nurses, state that confidentiality is paramount and that disclosure can only be made with consent (United Kingdom Central Council for Nursing, Midwifery and Health Visiting, 1992). Accordingly, in such cases, possible constraints to the counselling process which may result from concerns over confidentiality should not occur, and patients should be made aware of the confidential nature of any counselling session.

Such confidentiality should form part of a contract made with patients. Here, a contract does not mean a written and signed piece of paper. Instead, in providing care, be it emotional, informational or counselling, the helper makes a verbal, but explicit, contract with the person involved. This may simply be a statement of the confidentiality about what is said. It may also involve an agreement to meet again at an agreed time. As counselling is based on trust between helper and client, it is crucial that such contracts are honoured wherever possible, and that reasonable explanations are given if they cannot be.

A Problem-solving Approach to Counselling

Egan identifies three distinct and interrelated stages in the helping process. These logically follow from each other, with the success of each successive stage relying on that of the previous one. These three stages are briefly described below, before examining the skills required to negotiate each stage in more detail.

Stage 1: Problem exploration and clarification. Here, the goal of counselling is to help the person identify their problems. This may sound very simple, but is not always so. Many people may be unaware, for example, of exactly why they are unhappy or why they are failing to cope. A person may report that they always seem to be miserable and lethargic, and seem to spend all their time moping about the house feeling sorry for themselves. Whilst this is an accurate description of the problem at one level, it provides little basis for identifying a solution and changing the situation. If the person can explore the reasons *why* they are feeling this way, they may be better able to do something to help themselves. For example, they may feel this way because they do not feel able to visit their friends as frequently as they could before their MI.

Stage 2: Goal-setting. Once a problem has been defined, it is more easily resolved. The second stage in problem resolution, therefore, is to determine what needs to be done to resolve the problem: to establish a reasonable goal or subgoals. Using the previous example, the person may set a goal of seeing their friends more often. Note that they need not identify how their goals should be achieved at this stage, they simply need to clarify what those goals are. In some cases, subgoals can be set which move the person towards a final target. For example, if someone is trying to lose weight they may set subgoals of achieving so much weight loss per week, as well as a larger, longer-term, goal of trying to achieve a target weight.

Stage 3: Facilitating action. The final stage in the counselling process is for the person being counselled to identify ways in which their chosen goals, or subgoals, may be achieved and to facilitate the person in taking up these approaches. To identify methods of achieving goals often requires consideration of a number of alternative strategies before arriving at a final approach to put into action.

Of course, the counselling process does not necessarily proceed so smoothly and may loop back to a previous stage, or even miss stages out. Many people, for example, may feel that they need no further help after achieving a clearer understanding of their problems. Nevertheless, these stages provide a basic framework to the counselling process; it is important to be aware of where you are in the process, and not to rush or vacillate between stages. Before looking at the counselling process in more detail, a case example from a primary care setting may make these processes more explicit.

Case Study

Mrs T took part in a regular screening clinic held at her local general practitioner's surgery, where she was found to be obese and to have a raised serum cholesterol level. Following standard dietary advice, Mrs T agreed to a goal of losing two pounds of weight per week over the following months. She was given a leaflet providing standard information about the fat and calorific content of a variety of foods, and a leaflet detailing a number of 'healthy' recipes.

On follow-up visits, Mrs T's serum cholesterol and weight were unchanged and a psychologist was asked to see her. The psychologist began to explore why Mrs T had not responded to the advice given previously. Mrs T explained that she already knew which were 'healthy' or 'unhealthy' food choices. Indeed, she had been on many diets before, but without success. She felt she only had to 'look at food to put on weight'. Thus, up to this point goals had been set that were essentially unachievable.

The psychologist then began to explore in some detail with Mrs T why she was having difficulty losing weight. A number of problems became apparent. One important factor Mrs T identified was that she was not getting the support she needed from her family, and in particular from her grown-up sons. Mrs T was the family cook, in a family that often demanded 'fry-ups'. She accepted this role, but had difficulty not nibbling the food as she cooked it. Although she actually ate quite small (and low fat) meals, many of her calories came from nibbling while cooking.

Mrs T's husband supported her attempts to lose weight and was prepared to change his diet to help her. However, her sons, who both lived at the family home and had their own flats, often demanded meals late at night when they got back from the pub, usually hungry and the worse for drink. So Mrs T frequently started to cook late at night, at the end of what may have been a successful day of dieting. She then nibbled high calorie food while cooking, and ended the day on a negative note, which in turn, lowered her motivation to diet the following day, establishing a vicious circle of over-eating.

Once this very specific problem had been identified, Mrs T was able to establish a new subgoal that would potentially help her to achieve her main one of losing weight. After some discussion with the psychologist, she felt that as both her sons were adults it was inappropriate that they arrive late at night and demand that she cook for them. In future, if they wanted to eat, they would have to cook it themselves! Mrs T therefore established the goal of not cooking their late night meals.

Once the goal was established, Mrs T felt a little concerned about how her sons would react to her no longer cooking for them. The next part of the counselling session was therefore spent deciding how she should best set about telling them. She finally decided that she would tell them in the coming week, explaining why she felt she could no longer cook for them at the time of night they were demanding food. She even rehearsed what she would say to them.

This story shows how problem-solving counselling works. An initial goal was set (lose two pounds of weight each week), which proved difficult to achieve. In response, Mrs T was encouraged to identify what was preventing this from happening. Once identified, a further goal was set and ways of achieving it explored.

This story also illustrates the dangers of assuming that simply providing people with information about what to do, in this case to lose weight, is sufficient. Some people will successfully act upon information that is given. Others, for a variety of reasons, will not. If the latter is the case, it is important that the professionals' responses are not simply exasperation and repetition of information (which they typically are), but that wherever possible some attempt is made to find out *why* a goal has not been achieved, and to find ways of facilitating appropriate change.

We can now look in more detail at the skills needed to negotiate each stage.

Stage 1: Problem exploration and clarification

The main goal of the first stage of counselling is to identify in some detail the problems a person is facing, and to determine which of these they may wish to change.

The main skills of the helper in this phase are listening and eliciting the information required to help both helper and patient to gain an accurate representation of the problems they face. This may not always be as simple as it sounds. The person may be overwhelmed by problems they are aware of, but feel powerless to do anything about; they may feel powerful emotions such as sadness, anger, or depression but may be unable to pinpoint their cause.

The goal of counselling in each of these cases is to facilitate the individual's identification and understanding of the cause or causes of their distress that may be amenable to change; and to move from large insoluble problems to smaller potentially solvable problems. More articulate people may be able to achieve this with minimal help from a helper. However, this is by no means always the case, and a number of skills may be used to encourage problem exploration, such as:

- direct questioning and prompts;
- silence and minimal prompts;
- empathic feedback;
- the 'puzzled detective'.

Direct questioning and prompts. The simplest way of encouraging individuals to explore relevant issues is to ask them direct questions about the problems they are experiencing: 'Why did you . . .?', 'How did it feel when you . . .?', 'What happened after . . .?', and so on. This approach may provide a good understanding of the problems a person is facing, particularly if 'open' questions, which encourage exploration of issues are used. The opposite of this style, using closed questions which encourage one word answers ('Yes', 'No') will be less useful.

The information asked for should be as specific as possible. Vague questions get vague answers, and do not help specify problems in sufficient detail so that specific solutions can be identified. If problems appear diffuse and apparently all-pervading, it may be necessary to explore a number of specific aspects or representative examples. A full understanding of a person's problems involves exploration of their:

- experiences: what happened to them;
- their behaviour: what they did in response;
- their feelings and emotions associated with these events.

The judicious use of direct questioning can be used to explore each of these. However, too many questions may make the person feel they are being grilled, and interfere with the development or maintenance of rapport. Accordingly, alternative methods of exploration may be useful.

A second direct method of problem exploration is equally simple and takes the form of prompts and probes requesting information: for example, 'Tell me about . . .', 'Describe to me how you felt about . . .', and so on.

The use of direct questions, prompts and focusing on particular episodes is shown in the case of Mr B who saw a helper after having experienced problems following discharge from hospital. Mr B had begun to experience frequent feelings of panic with angina-like symptoms. These episodes occurred at home and work and Mr B had previously been unable to point to any particular reason for these episodes. They just seemed to happen 'out of the blue':

Helper: *Could you tell me a little about the problems you're experiencing?*

Mr B: *Yes. I'm not really sure where to start. I seem to be having lots of 'funny turns'. I feel a tremendous pain across my chest and get sweaty and panicky.*

My doctor says they're nothing to worry about, but they're really quite frightening.

Helper: *How often do you get these feelings?*

Mr B: *Quite often. About once a day. Sometimes at work, sometimes at home.*

The helper now has some idea of the extent of the problem. Together, they begin to find out in more detail what happens when Mr B has these panic attacks.

Helper: *I'm beginning to get some understanding of the problem. It may help me get a better picture of what's happening if you could describe in a bit more detail one particular time when you felt this way. Can you think back to a recent time?*

Mr B: *OK. I had one this morning before I came to you.*

Helper: *Tell me what happened then.*

Mr B: *Well, I was getting ready to come to the hospital. I was in the lounge, and I began to feel a pain in my chest, and my hands started shaking and I was sweating. I became a bit panicky and shaky . . .*

Helper: *I see. What did you do when you felt these symptoms?*

Mr B: *Well, I was fighting for my breath, so I had to sit down and breathe deeply until they began to go away.*

Helper: *How long did that take?*

Mr B: *Only a few minutes, but that was enough. It feels awful.*

Helper: *I'm beginning to get a better understanding of what happens to you now. But I'm still not clear what seems to be setting these turns off in the first place. Can you think of anything that may have triggered the one you had this morning?*

Mr B: *Not really. As I say, they just seem to come out of the blue.*

Helper: *I've seen people before with similar problems to this. Sometimes their episodes were triggered by stress or by exertion. I wonder whether there was anything on your mind this morning, or if you had been pushing yourself a little.*

Mr B: *It's funny you should say that. I was a bit worried about coming to see you today. That was preying on my mind. I didn't know what to expect. I suppose that may have got me going today . . .*

Now the helper acts on a hunch, and tries to identify a common cause linking all these episodes:

Helper: *I wonder if worries or stress may have triggered some of the other attacks you've had . . . ?*

Mr B: *I wonder . . . ? I suppose I am quite a 'nervy' type of person. I do get uptight about things . . .*

In order to show how a line of questioning may develop, this dialogue was shortened from the original version. More time may have usefully been spent in exploring some of the issues raised. For example, it would have been important to find out exactly in which order Mr B's symptoms occurred. If he felt the chest pain before any other symptoms this may suggest that he is overreacting to an episode of angina. If any pain followed the other symptoms, this may suggest that he is having panic attacks which are resulting in, among other things, an episode of angina. The way these are tackled in the problem resolution stage may be quite different.

This direct approach to problem exploration can be very demanding of people, and care needs to be taken to ensure that this is not the only exploratory technique used. Rather less active and demanding methods of problem exploration need to be built in as well. The first of these may simply be silence.

Silence and minimal prompts. Because of their very nature, many issues explored in counselling sessions have not been thought through by patients. If they had, counselling may be unnecessary. Because of this, the process should not be rushed; if there is a silence, this need not necessarily be filled by the helper. The person may simply need time to think through a problem or consider a point. Accordingly, one way of facilitating problems is to allow, or even encourage, pauses and time for thought, and not to continually bombard people with requests for information. If patients pause, and seem to have more to say, the use of minimal prompts such as 'mmm' or 'uh-huh' may also be a powerful way of encouraging exploration:

Patient: *I was rather shocked when I was told I had high blood pressure . . .*

Helper: *Uh-huh.*

Patient: *Yes . . . my first worry was that . . .*

Empathic feedback. Another method of gaining information is through the use of empathic feedback. Reflecting back an understanding of the person's situation and their feelings can be powerful encouragement in helping the individual explore their problems, frequently more often than a direct question. If nothing else, it will give feedback to the helper as to whether they are truly understanding their patient.

Returning to the example of Mr B, some of his feelings at the time of his panic attacks could have been explored through empathic feedback. For example, he hinted at how anxious he felt at the time of these episodes:

Mr B: *Well, I was fighting for my breath, so I had to sit down and breathe deeply until they began to go away.*

Helper: *How long did that take?*

Mr B: *Only a few minutes, but that was enough. It feels awful.*

An empathic statement, such as *'It sounds as if these attacks really make you feel quite scared . . .'* may have elicited more information about how Mr B felt at these times.

Empathic feedback can show the patient the helper's understanding of their situation and their feelings. This in itself may promote exploration of a problem more than a direct question. Finally, it can provide important feedback to the helper as to whether they are truly understanding their patients.

Egan identified a number of ways by which helpers may develop more accurate empathy. First, by giving themselves time to think. All helpers, however skilled, need time to think about what the person has said, and to reflect this back to them. Patients may not always give helpers this time, and move rapidly on without pause. In this case, helpers should make time by interrupting the flow by either verbal or non-verbal signs ('Let me see if I've got what you're saying . . .'). Empathic responses should be reasonably frequent, but also short and to the point. They should also match the language and tone of voice of the patient.

The 'puzzled detective'. If patients are forthcoming with information, problem exploration using a variety of these techniques is often straightforward. More difficult are sessions where patients volunteer little information or information that is confused and confusing. One way round this is the 'puzzled detective' routine. In this, the helper takes responsibility for any problem clarification, and in so doing, reduces any feelings of inadequacy or frustration that the patient may experience resulting from such a communication problem:

Helper: *I'm being a bit slow here . . . Could you just run through that again, so I get a better picture of exactly what happened?*

Helper: *I'm beginning to understand how frightening the experience of these panicky episodes can be, but I'm still not sure what made you panic last week at work.*

Of course, such an approach should be used carefully. Over-use may be distracting and make the *helper* appear inept.

It is worth reiterating that the primary goal of counselling at this stage is to help the patient explore issues *relevant* to their problems; it is not to gather information for its own sake. This is not only ethically questionable, but it can distract from effective exploration of the problem. Relevant information is generally in the here-and-now, and is either problem-related or solution-oriented. The goal is to achieve appropriate disclosure of information with the least prompting and effort from the helper. Too much prompting will make a patient feel cajoled and less powerful than the helper. This may have the effect of not empowering them to identify their own solutions to their problems.

Egan suggests two rules of thumb to make sure that this situation does not arise: first, after having probed or prompted a response from a patient, the helper should let the patient take the initiative in exploring the information it yields; second, after using a probe, use empathy rather than another probe or series of probes as a way of encouraging further exploration.

Stage 2: Goal-setting

The primary aim of this stage is to help the patient begin to identify ways in which to manage or resolve the problems that have been identified in the problem exploration stage: that is, to set clearly delineated goals by which such changes may be brought about. In this case, a goal is a clear, concrete, statement of what a person intends to do, spelled out in precise terms ('I will join an exercise class', not 'I must try to get more fit.'). A goal should be precise and manageable.

Achieving goals can encourage further progress; failure can exacerbate the problem: 'I tried – and failed. It shows how impossible my problems are to resolve'. For this reason, it is important to ensure that goals are realistic in terms of the patient's resources, and social and environmental situation. They should also be consonant with their values and lifestyle. For example, it may be inappropriate to establish a goal of exercising five times a week if the person has previously been a 'couch potato'. They may find such a demanding goal inappropriate and lack motivation to achieve it. Where a goal is difficult to achieve immediately, a series of subgoals may be established.

Typical concrete goals might be: 'I will have an overall goal of jogging three times a week, for at least 20 minutes on each occasion. I will build up gradually. In the first week I will walk briskly for 10 minutes; 'I will lose two pounds of weight a week until I reach my target weight'; or, 'I will put aside at least 20 minutes each day to play with my kids'. These may be compared with rather less concrete goals of: 'I'd better do some more exercise'; 'I'll try to lose some weight over the next few weeks'; and, 'I'd like to put some time aside to be with my kids more'. The first goals are both achievable and clear. They allow progress to be monitored, and successes and failures noted when the time comes to put them into action. Some goals may become clear immediately following the problem exploration phase:

Mr H: *I must admit I was shocked when I got the cholesterol results. I thought I led a quite healthy life. Not superfit; but not seriously unfit. But now we've discussed some of the things that have led to this I think I can begin to think of ways I could improve without too much effort. I could begin to . . .*

Patient: (who has become over dependent on his wife): *Gosh! Now I've actually spelled out what I've been doing I'm embarrassed by it all! My poor wife has been running after me all day, and I've let her. Even small jobs I could easily do, I've begun to depend on her to do . . . And then I take my boredom and frustration out on her, she loses her temper, and gets me uptight, and off we go! I guess there are some things I could do to take something off her plate, and they may even help me not to be so down in the dumps . . .*

However, not all patients will see the way out of their problems even after they have been fully explored. Despite a fuller understanding, they may be locked into old ways of looking at things, and not be able to adopt a differing and possibly more effective viewpoint.

In order to achieve this, the perspective of the counselling process now begins to change. In the first stage of counselling, the goal is to explore issues from the patient's perspective. The second phase involves helping them to explore their problem from a new perspective, which enables them to decide what to do to resolve their problems: to set goals for change.

Because goal-setting is not always the clear and easy task it may appear to be, a number of skills and tactics have been identified which may be useful at this stage in the counselling process. These include:

- summarizing;
- providing relevant information;
- challenging, to identify new perspectives.

Summarizing. At some stage, the counselling process moves from problem exploration to attempts at problem resolution. This change may be initiated by the patient, as in the examples above. Even if a good understanding of the problems has been achieved but they do not begin to look for ways of dealing with them, the helper may have to make this transition clear. This can best be achieved by summarizing the important elements of the situation, ensuring that both they and the patient have the same understanding of the issues.

A good summary involves pulling together the *relevant* material. This focusing may in itself move patients from exploration to trying to think of ways of dealing with a problem. If not, it may be necessary to invite or suggest that now is the time to explore ways of dealing with them:

Helper: *Let's look at what we've got so far. You've told me about a number of things which may be contributing to your weight problem. You find it difficult to avoid snacks, and often eat fried food. You also don't exercise as much as you used to, something which you used to enjoy . . .*

Mr D: *Yes. I suppose that's about it. Just listening to you, it seems there are two things I'd like to get to grips with. First I need to avoid some of the snacks that I'm having; although quite how I'm not sure. I'd also like to do something about this exercise business. I really did enjoy exercise. I think if I took it up again, it may help motivate me to keep my eating down.*

Providing information. Sometimes patients cannot explore problem situations fully because they lack information. This is particularly pertinent for those facing challenges and problems they have not encountered before, either directly or indirectly. Problems in rehabilitation often prove to be such instances: 'How much exercise is reasonable to take after an MI?'; 'When is it reasonable to go out shopping without someone with you?'.

People may be stuck in ruts, depressed, frightened of doing too much, yet feeling frustrated at their inactivity, partly because of inappropriate fears and anxieties. The simple provision of information about what to expect, and what other people with similar degrees of cardiac damage are doing may be helpful in guiding patients toward a reasonable course of action.

Mr A: *It's OK for my wife to say I should be getting back into my old routines. But I don't know what I can do! Can I carry heavy bags, play sport? I'd like to do some of these things — just to get her off my back!*

Helper: *It may be worth me giving you some idea about what you might reasonably be able to do. Let me tell you what some other people with a similar heart attack to yours get up to after a few months at home . . .*

Challenges. When patients feel unable to identify any goals, or feel little can be done to change a situation, such ways of thinking may require challenging by the helper. This does not mean confrontation: the skills of challenging are used to help people to explore their problems and potential solutions from new perspectives. Several types of challenge can be identified, including:

- invitations to explore solutions;
- challenging of assumptions;
- direct challenge;
- identification of possibilities.

The first type of challenging may be as an *invitation* to explore new ideas and identify new goals. Direct and forthright challenging of their pre-existing views and ideas may simply alienate patients, and result in them withdrawing from the counselling process. The example below involves some problem exploration using primary empathy, before the helper invites the patient to explore some possible goals in an attempt to resolve his problems.

Helper: *So, after these anger outbursts, you feel upset and confused . . .*

Mr C: *Yes, because I don't really know what triggers these things in the first place. If there was one thing which would make me feel happier, and my wife as well, it would be to lessen this tension and anger I feel . . .*

Helper: *I wonder if after you've been angry you've ever thought about how you could have avoided feeling that way in the first place . . .*

Mr C: *No! But perhaps I ought to. Hey, that may be part of the problem itself! I just react and let fly without really thinking about things. Come to think of it, when I get angry it's not really about the thing which has just happened. I've usually been bottling it up for some time before I blow.*

Helper: *Perhaps it may be useful to look at these things which get you bottled up . . .*

Mr C (after some thought): *Do you know, I think the worst thing is the frustration I feel about not doing anything: not contributing to the finances, not working any more. I just sit around the house and brood. The thoughts just take over and I get angry with myself, then something happens and kaboom! Off I go!*

More direct challenging may sometimes be necessary, for example, if a person is stuck with a negative and self-deafeating view of their problems, and is unwilling to think about potential solutions. They may attribute their depression to a personal failure to cope with their problems, and feel this is likely to be a continuing state of affairs because they are inadequate and generally do not cope well. If not challenged, this type of internal dialogue can rapidly become a self-fulfilling prophesy. A helper may usefully provide an alternative perspective:

Helper: *I know you have these feelings, but I'm not sure this is the only conclusion that can be drawn. Given the shock of what has happened to you over the last few weeks, are you surprised you feel somewhat low? I know I would. But does this necessarily mean you have to feel this way in the future?*

A direct challenge may also be necessary if other approaches lead to simply going round in circles, or patients appear to be avoiding certain issues, providing discordant accounts of their feelings and behaviours. Direct challenges must always be delivered carefully and not so directly that the patient has no space to move:

Helper: *I'm getting a little confused here. I'd appreciate it if you'd help me out. Sometimes you seem to be saying to me that the problem lies with your marriage. It's been rocky for a number of years and there is little you can do about it. At other times you suggest the root of your anger is your frustration following your heart attack. I guess the problem may be a bit of both, but which is the most important?*

Helper: *Hang on a minute. First you say it's your marriage that's the problem, then it's your heart attack. Which is it?*

While both approaches challenge apparent discrepancies or distortions in the patient's description of events, the former does so more subtly, and does not force the patient into what could be an embarrassing attempt to wriggle around an issue rather than explore it more fully, without which identification of appropriate goals would be impossible.

Good challenging should test the strengths of the person, not their weaknesses. They should help them see what positive behaviours can take the place of negative ones. Finally, challenging will not be effective during the early stages of counselling: to be effective, the helper must have established good rapport, trust, and mutual respect with the client first.

Sometimes the problem in identifying a goal is the number of options open to the patient, and it may be necessary to explore which of these is preferred. From a patient's description of their problems it is often possible to identify a number of alternative strategies of change. It can sometimes be helpful to highlight the possibilities.

Mrs D: *I know that my anger stems from frustration and boredom and that I take it out on my family . . .*

Helper: *I guess this leaves you at least two alternative actions. First, you could look at ways of dealing with the anger when you feel you want to explode. Second, we could explore ways that may reduce these feelings of frustration you have.*

Stage 3: Facilitating action

Although goals have been established in the second counselling phase, patients may not yet have thought through how these may be achieved. Some people are able to mobilize their resources and achieve their goals without further help; others, who although they now have a good understanding of what the problem situation is and where they wish to move to, may still not have a clear idea of how to achieve the goals they have identified.

While the way in which some goals can best be achieved may be fairly obvious, sometimes this is not the case, or there may be so many potential ways that patients cannot see the wood for the trees. For example, the simple goal of going out twice a week could be achieved by visiting friends, watching sport, going to the pub, listening to live music, walking in the country, and so on. If a person wishes to control their anger or frustration, the list of methods of achieving this could be using relaxation techniques, distracting their attention from what is getting them angry, leaving the room or trying to see the humour in the situation. They may think about ways of reducing their background levels of frustration, if these are contributing to them getting angry by, for example, taking up a new hobby, going out more frequently (back to the previous list!), taking a part-time job, working more around the house, or beginning to exercise.

Brainstorming and the balance sheet. Brainstorming and the use of a balance sheet are powerful methods of helping people to identify possible ways of achieving goals, and deciding which of these is the best to use. Brainstorming gives the person time to think of as many possible ways of achieving their goals as is possible. To encourage brainstorming it is important to stress quantity, while suspending judgement on ideas:

Helper: *Be as adventurous or crazy as you like – we can sort out the sensible suggestions later. Who knows, some of the crazy suggestions may not appear so crazy at the end.*

Once a number of possibilities have been identified, the balance sheet can be an effective aid to decision making. This focuses on the utility and acceptability of following various alternative approaches to achieving goals. It can be done formally by writing the costs and benefits on a piece of paper and weighing the strengths and weaknesses of various courses of action, or informally through discussion. As in choosing goals, the route towards these goals must be concrete and specific, realistic, adequate, and in keeping with the person's values. They must also have a clear time-frame in which they should be accomplished.

At this point many people may feel they need no more help. They have identified new goals and how these can best be achieved. It is now up to them to carry them out. However, some people who have difficult goals to achieve may wish to have continued support while they try to put these plans into action. Frequently, this may involve repeated counselling sessions, in which the process of counselling essentially replicates that already described. Following each session, patients will have a clear goal or subgoal to achieve in the following week or weeks. Each subsequent session should examine whether the goal has been achieved, and if not, why not. Was it an inappropriate goal? Were there unseen problems? If so, goals may be changed or problems thought through. Patient and helper adopt a problem-solving approach, which deals with problems as they arise, but which keeps progression to an end goal as its primary objective.

One potential issue in the final stage of counselling is the need for skills training. People may require some help in achieving the goals they set. For example, people wishing to control feelings of stress or anger or giving up smoking may benefit from instruction in techniques or strategies to help them. Some of these are explored in the following two chapters.

Summary

The model of counselling developed by Egan comprises three stages: problem exploration and clarification, goal setting, and facilitating action.

❑ Problem exploration: the primary goal of this stage is to help the person achieve a clear and specific understanding of what their problems are. The helper may use the following skills to achieve this:

– direct questioning and prompts;
– the use of silence and minimal prompts;
– empathic feedback;
– the 'puzzled detective' routine.

❑ Goal setting: the aim is to determine what needs to be done to resolve the problem: to establish a goal or goals. These should be concrete, precise, and realistic. Tactics which may be used to help people define goals include summarizing, providing relevant information, and challenging. Types of challenge include:

– invitations to explore solutions;
– challenging assumptions;
– direct challenge;
– identification of possibilities.

❑ Action: this involves helping the person to identify ways of achieving their goals and, if necessary, facilitating in taking up these approaches. Two strategies involve brainstorming and use of a balance sheet.

4

Stress Management Training

Mr S: *Last week we agreed that I would try to do more exercise. We agreed that I would have a long-term goal of exercising three times a week for 20 minutes, and could try to achieve that goal in stages. My goal for the week was to walk briskly for 10 minutes on two days during the week. The problem is that every time I try to exercise I just get worried . . . more than worried, I get panicky. I worry that I'm going to set off my symptoms again and that I could have another heart attack. This sounds silly talking to you now, but once I start exercising and I begin to feel my heart pounding, I panic and just have to stop. I can't think of any way that I can achieve these goals.*

While the model of counselling described so far provides a useful framework to the counselling process, it has a number of limitations. In particular, while it allows patients to develop a clear understanding of their problems, and the changes they wish to make, it does not necessarily empower them to make these changes. Patients may not have the skills or resources to do so. For this reason, Egan saw his basic framework as being able to integrate a number of adjunctive counselling and skills-based interventions. This chapter focuses on teaching techniques known as stress management skills, which can be used by patients to help them cope with stress, anxiety, or depression.

Stress management techniques can help patients to modify negative mood states and any consequent problems of rehabilitation. They may be used to help manage angina, particularly for those people who experience it at times of stress or strong emotions. They may also be of benefit to people with generally stressful lives, even if they do not experience negative feelings as a result of that stress, which may still influence their risk of re-infarction (see Chapter 5). Stress management may also form part of a preventive programme, for example, teaching stress management techniques to people found to have raised blood pressure or cholesterol as part of a multi-disciplinary intervention.

A Model of Stress

Lazarus and Folkman (1984) suggest that stress results from a disparity between the perceived *demands* made of an individual and their perceived *ability to cope* with them. In the first stage of this process, known as primary appraisal, the person evaluates the situation in terms of whether it may result in some negative consequences. In the second stage, known as secondary appraisal, the person assesses the resources they can use to deal with the situation. If demands are high, and the person's perceived ability to cope is also high, they will not feel stressed. Thus, for example, the archetypal stressed executive may not experience stress: although the demands placed on them may be high, most executives feel able to cope with them. Indeed, many thrive on meeting the challenges they provide. They, and any other person, will only experience stress when they feel they cannot cope effectively. However, if the demands made of a person (at whatever level) exceed their perceived ability to meet them, they come under stress; that is, they experience stressful cognitions (thoughts), emotions and physiological responses.

Triggers to stress. We tend to think of stress as a response to major events in our lives, such as divorce or job loss. Although these can have a major impact on our lives, and have been shown to trigger illness, depression, and so on, it is the less dramatic hassles which probably do the most damage. Over-reacting to these frequent triggers can facilitate the disease process, and for those who already have manifest CHD, lead to further risk of infarction or episodes of angina. Triggers need not necessarily be external events: worrying about problems may trigger stressful emotional, physiological, and behavioural responses.

Some triggers to stress, as in the case of Mr S, are obvious. Others are less so. Typical triggers that many of us deal with in our daily lives are waiting in queues, arguing with a partner, dealing with fractious children, or working to tight deadlines. Because these hassles are so frequent and part of our everyday lives, we often do not think of them as being particularly stressful. Yet their relative frequency means they may contribute to a variety of stress symptoms, varying from irritability to feelings of emotional or physical exhaustion.

Responses to stress

Cognitive responses. It is possible to imagine how our thoughts may either increase or decrease stress and affect both our emotions and level of physical tension. For example, imagine you are stuck in a traffic jam and already late for an appointment. You are unlikely to be able to relax if your thoughts are screaming 'Hurry up! This is a disaster. I'm going to be very late . . .' 'What the *&^%! is holding this $#%! queue up!' All such thoughts do is exacerbate the stress process, and make relaxation difficult, if not impossible. If your thoughts follow a different line, 'Well, there's nothing I can do about this, I may as well relax and make the most of it', 'If I'm late, its not that much of a problem', relaxation and emotional control will be easier, or even unnecessary.

People do not go round talking to themselves – at least not all the time! Instead, we often behave in an apparently 'thought-less' fashion. This is not to say that such thoughts do not occur. Instead they are mainly automatic, very quick, and are often unconscious. Nevertheless, they may profoundly alter our mood and stress levels. Take, for example, Mr W:

Case Study

Mr W was a single man in his thirties who had experienced some chest pain while weight-lifting. He had initially ignored his symptoms, but the pain had increased and he had soon felt close to collapse. He reported these symptoms to the staff at the health club, and they called an ambulance. On admission to the local hospital, Mr W was diagnosed as having had an MI, and was admitted to CCU.

After an uncomplicated period in CCU, Mr W was transferred to a general medical ward. While there, he appeared, to some, to be a model patient, being quiet and making no particular demands on the nursing or medical staff. However, although there were several young men on the ward, Mr W did not mix with them, spending most of the day by his bed, and ignoring the television or company in the day room. His appetite was poor, and, although he was able to raise a smile when talked to, it seemed a little forced. The physiotherapist found Mr W to be anxious during his rehabilitation exercises, and he was making poor progress in the graded programme she was trying to implement.

One member of staff spent some time talking to Mr W. It emerged that he felt both anxious and depressed. Until his admission he had thought of himself as a fit and healthy person. He went to a health club regularly, and although he knew he was slightly overweight he thought this was compensated for by his exercise and lifestyle. The MI had had a profound impact on Mr W's thoughts about his health and his self-image, which were both catastrophic and self-defeating. For example: 'I've had a heart attack! Jeez, I'm only 34! That's really bad! This must mean I'm really unfit and my health is shot. When's the next one going to come? . . . That could be it. Am I going to die?' Another train of thought he would slip into was slightly more positive, in that he assumed he would resume some sort of life again. But again, Mr W saw his future life to be profoundly and adversely affected by his MI: 'Even if I do live, this heart disease is going to mess things up . . . It's not as if me and the boss get on well . . . I'm going to need time off to recover . . . That could be it . . . He won't like that. I could be fired! And what about my social life? I won't have any money. But what would I need that for anyway, I'm hardly going to be going out much any more with the boys . . .'

Mr W was reluctant to exercise because of a fear of triggering chest pain, which he was continuing to have occasionally. The pain triggered memories and fears he had felt during the MI, and he feared the pain heralded a further MI: 'Oh, no! My chest hurts again . . . I'm not getting better . . . If I push myself it's going to hurt more . . . I can't do anything right . . . If I exercise it hurts, and that can't be right. If I don't exercise, then I'm never going to get better'.

Mr W may appear to be progressing well, if slowly; however, his thought processes reflected a high degree of depressive thinking, which, unless they were challenged were likely to have a profound and deleterious effect on his rehabilitation. Such thoughts may never have become apparent if someone had not sat down with Mr W to discuss how he was feeling.

A minority of people do not find the rehabilitation process threatening or potentially stressful; they may have absolute faith in the doctors' ability to cure them; they may think that having survived their initial MI that they will inevitably get better; or have a religious faith that helps them to cope. However, most people will find the process somewhat stressful. While relieved to have survived their MI, they will be worried about their future health and its consequences to themselves and their family. Thus, the primary appraisal may well be, 'There's something to worry about here . . .'

The degree of stress they experience will be modified by how well they think they can cope with rehabilitation. Some people, who perhaps know someone who has made a good recovery from MI or who are generally 'good copers', may be confident in their ability to deal with the problems they will encounter, and experience little stress. Others may be less confident and experience more stress. It is this latter group, those who are both anxious about their future and how they will cope, who are likely to have the most problems during rehabilitation.

Emotional responses. If a person fails to cope adequately with the demands stemming from the stress trigger, they may experience a whole gamut of emotions, varying from anger or irritability to anxiety or depression. If stresses continue for a long period, such as coping with a long and difficult period of rehabilitation, this may lead to profound feelings of depression and helplessness.

Physiological responses. Alongside these psychological responses to stress are a number of physiological ones. In the short-term, these are characterized by the so-called 'flight or fight' response. In this, the sympathetic nervous system responds to trigger events by rapidly increasing heart rate and blood pressure, and by releasing free fatty acids into the bloodstream to enable a fast physical response to any event. If the trigger does not require such a strong physical reaction, the result is an increased, and inappropriate, stress on the heart, and the conversion of unused free fatty acids by the liver into cholesterol, thus exacerbating the disease process. Acute stress may also trigger an angina attack by increasing the heart muscle's requirement for oxygen, at the same time as causing mild vaso-spasm of the coronary arteries, resulting in the transient ischaemia typical of angina.

Essentially, we each have a nervous system that is designed to deal with Stone Age crises (such as meeting a sabre-toothed tiger while out for an afternoon stroll) which demand rapid physical action (run like hell!) in an age when most stresses are psychological in nature and do not require physical action.

Unless we learn ways to moderate such responses, there is a gradual wearing down of the body's resources and the development of disease processes. Thankfully, we have one means at our disposal to do this: a key marker to the degree of physiological arousal we are experiencing is the level of physical tension. The degree of physical tension in the skeletal muscles is partially mediated by sympathetic activity; the more physically tense you are, the greater the degree of physiological arousal.

This relationship between muscular tension and physiological arousal can be used to advantage in stress management. Relaxation procedures can be used to consciously moderate levels of physical tension, providing negative feedback to the sympathetic nervous system, and serving to dampen down the flight or fight response.

Behavioural responses. What do you do when you lose your keys? I often ask this question in workshops to teach stress-management skills. The response is typically a number of rather embarrassed smiles.

Most people admit to doing rather silly and illogical things. They search their pockets and, having done so and failed to find their keys, almost immediately search them again; a behaviour totally without logic! Even minor stresses can result in illogical and stressed behaviour. Short-term stress may result in panic or angry behaviour. Longer-term responses to stress may involve increased consumption of drugs, like cigarettes and alcohol, to help maintain an equilibrium or to avoid the cause of the stress. This latter tactic may work in the short term; for example, Mr S (page 52) would reduce or even abolish his stress by avoiding exercise. However, the long-term consequences may be less positive.

It should be noted that stress does not simply stem from the environment as a one-way process. Often, stressed individuals inadvertently create and engender reactions in others that maintain maladaptive stress responses: the behaviour which is intended to solve problems often ends up intensifying them. For example, people frightened of over-exerting themselves may elicit over-protectiveness in others, which may serve to further invalid them, confirm their anxieties, and lead them to seek further over-protectiveness, strengthening the vicious cycle.

Some Implications for Stress Management

An implication of the model described here is that stress is not an event which happens out of the blue. It is a *process*, involving both external events and a variety of internal reactions to these events. Changes to any part of this process will alter the degree of stress experienced. Stress management strategies may focus on changing triggers, changing thoughts about these triggers, or changing physiological or behavioural responses to such thoughts or triggers. In doing so, the negative emotions related to stress will also be moderated.

Stress management comprises a whole gamut of techniques ranging from relaxation to assertiveness training. Not all are appropriate to all patients – the differing problems facing patients require different coping strategies. In addition, patients have differing aptitudes and capabilities, and find some techniques easier to master than others. It is therefore important that the introduction and choice of techniques stems from a collaboration between patient and helper, and that interventions are tailored to the individual's situations and capabilities. Even so, while most patients will readily be able to learn and use relaxation techniques, some may find the cognitive, or thought, strategies described below not so easy to implement.

As its name implies, the primary goal of stress management is not to encourage patients to eliminate stress, which would make life very boring! Instead, the goal of training is to ensure that patients have a variety of skills to help them cope with – that is, manage – stress constructively.

Stress management and the Egan model

Stress management skills should not be seen as separate to the Egan model of counselling (Chapter 3). Identifying whether or not they are necessary to help a patient involves the same process of problem-identification and goal-setting as any other aspect of counselling.

Where they differ is in the final stage of counselling, the action stage. Here, specific skills training may be necessary to help people manage stress more effectively. This fits well into the Egan model. However, it has its dangers. There is the potential to move from a collaborative relationship to one of 'expert' and 'patient'. This may disempower some people and make them less innovative in their ways of dealing with their problems. It is, therefore, extremely important that the teaching and learning of these skills remains a collaborative venture between patient and counsellor, not simply a didactic teaching exercise.

Many people easily see the value of learning relaxation, although fewer see the importance of thinking in causing and minimizing stress. Accordingly, the rest of this chapter focuses on the mechanics of teaching relaxation skills, and examines in more detail how patients may be made more aware of the importance of their thought processes in mediating stress, as well as how these can be changed.

Relaxation

The first, and often only, stress management technique many counsellors teach is that of physical relaxation. This focuses on minimizing the physiological aspects of the stress response. In doing so it provides patients with a new coping strategy, and may change their thoughts and emotions when dealing with stress. If nothing else, concentrating on relaxation may interrupt any negative, stress-engendering thoughts a person is having.

Relaxation is relatively simple to learn and use. Some people may feel these skills are all they wish to learn; others may want to learn additional techniques. Either way, relaxation training provides a useful and effective method of helping to control stress. It can easily be taught to groups, making it a useful cost-effective intervention.

The aim of relaxation training is to help people to be as relaxed as possible, and is appropriate, throughout the day and particularly at times of potential stress. Although learning relaxation involves lying or sitting quietly for some minutes away from the hustle and bustle of everyday life, its ultimate value is its immediate application at times of potential stress. There is little value to be gained by becoming increasingly tense during the day and unwinding at night in a comfy chair. However expert someone may become at this sort of relaxation, it will have absolutely no effect on the impact of daily stress. Learning to use relaxation skills appropriately involves developing awareness of stress, as evidenced through physical tension, and learning how to minimize such tension. This is best achieved using three interacting approaches:

• learning relaxation skills;
• learning to identify and monitor tension in daily life;
• learning to use relaxation skills at times of stress.

Learning relaxation skills

Patients may come to learn relaxation through a variety of routes. Following problem-oriented counselling they may identify tension and stress as a particular problem, and a goal may be to learn skills to help them cope more effectively with it. More frequently, patients will be taught relaxation skills as part of a more general treatment package. The process of learning and using these skills is the same; only the way in which they are initially presented may differ.

Learning relaxation skills is best achieved in a number of stages. The first involves learning to relax under optimal conditions. At this stage the patient is led through the process of relaxation, initially by the counsellor, and then typically by repeated practice listening to a cassette tape of instructions at home. Practice can also be repeated in subsequent counselling sessions if this is felt appropriate by counsellor and patient. This decision will depend on the degree of progress made through home practice, the time available for counselling, and the need to discuss other issues.

Relaxation practice is best conducted where the patient can fully relax. This may be on a bed, a floor-mat, or a chair which supports the neck, shoulders, and arms. Full relaxation cannot be practised on ordinary chairs, since these do not provide sufficient support, and require some tension to avoid falling off. Patients may need to loosen tight clothing, take off shoes, or whatever is needed to feel comfortable. As in all counselling, privacy must be assured, and sufficient time allowed to ensure no interruptions.

Before going through the actual relaxation procedures, it is important to provide a rationale for relaxation and to prepare the patient for what is going to happen. Where they are obviously stressed and tense, the rationale may be obvious. However, where relaxation is taught as part of a standardized post-MI rehabilitation or preventive programme (see Chapter 6), its benefits may be less obvious – that is, until patients have experienced the pleasure of deep relaxation. (A detailed rationale and preparation for group relaxation can be found in Appendix A.)

The relaxation process can then begin (Appendix B describes this in detail). This involves working through the entire body, tensing and then relaxing groups of muscles. Each part of the body in turn is tensed slightly and then relaxed, twice. The aim is to teach the patient to recognize tension and then to relax it away. For this reason, the level of tension does not need to be great, and the emphasis should be on the relaxation aspect of the exercise. To ensure deep relaxation it is also important that these procedures are conducted in an unhurried way.

Relaxation can also be taught using a pre-recorded cassette tape. This has obvious benefits on a busy CCU or surgical ward, where patients can be given a relaxation tape to use on a personal stereo. In this way, they can practise relaxation at an early stage after MI or an operation with little use of nurse or other professionals' time and without embarrassment or disturbance of other patients. Ideally, at least the initial session should be guided by someone skilled in teaching relaxation techniques. It is amazing how what may seem perfectly clear instructions on tape become misinterpreted by listeners, who may engage in quite bizarre postures in an attempt to comply with the instructions! Such confusion can be prevented by someone being there to help and guide as necessary. Going through the relaxation procedures with the patient can help the counselling relationship to develop. Indeed, many patients like to tape record the original relaxation session and use this later to practise, mistakes, interruptions, and all! This also has the benefit that the relaxation instructions can be tailored to suit the needs of the individual person, for example, those who have difficulty completing the standard protocol, as in the case of those with arthritis.

In order to use relaxation skills effectively at times of stress, it is important that patients practise relaxation regularly. Many patients are therefore given either a pre-recorded relaxation tape or one made of the relaxation training. They may be asked to listen to this regularly (usually once a day) and practise at home. As in the counselling session, patients need to ensure they can practise without interruption and without time pressure. It does not matter when they practise, although I usually advise people not to use the tape just before they go to bed. Although this may be a convenient time, its use at this time of night is more as a help to get off to sleep, not as the first stage of learning a skill to be used at any time of day.

When people become more skilled at relaxation – after, say, two or three weeks – the relaxation process can be speeded up by practising or using on tape an abbreviated form of instructions which miss out the tension part of the relaxation instructions, concentrating solely on those for relaxation.

Monitoring physical tension. At the same time as learning relaxation, patients can learn to monitor the times when they become physically tense in their daily lives. There are generally two sorts of situations to monitor. The first is during times of obvious problems, when the patient is aware they are feeling tense, for example when they feel angry, frustrated or anxious. The second level of tension is less easy to identify. This is the excess tension associated with everyday occurrences, such as dealing with queues, mild irritations during the day, or coping with demanding jobs. Here, the tension may be less obvious. People may have lived with this type of tension for many years and become used to it, treating it as normal. Yet continuous excess tension throughout the day can be tiring and, to someone with CHD, ultimately debilitating.

The first goal of monitoring physical tension is to learn to recognize when each sort of tension arises, and if possible what causes it. This can be achieved by teaching patients to monitor their level of physical tension at various times through the day. Many teachers of stress management skills formalize this learning process by asking patients to keep a 'tension diary'. This involves rating tension on a scale of, say, nought to ten, where nought means no tension at all and ten means the most tension possible. Patients can record their level of tension, say, every hour, or at key times during the day.

For each tension rating, a record may also be kept of its trigger. This may help in working on ways of reducing stress in the future. For example, if always working to self-imposed deadlines causes tension, at least two strategies for change may be appropriate: first, to try to relax at such times; secondly, to change the number of deadlines set.

For the first week or so, the diary can be used to record tension ratings alone. Later, it can be used to monitor patients' use of relaxation in their attempts to deal with their tension. An example of both types of diary is given in Figures 1 and 2.

WEDNESDAY		
Time	Level of tension (0–10)	Trigger
10.00	5	Just working hard
11.00	2	Relaxing during coffee break
12.00	4	Normal tension of work
13.00	8	Annoyed – had to work lunch break

Figure 1: Relaxation diary recording tension ratings

WEDNESDAY		
Level of tension (0–10)	Trigger	How successful (0–10)
6	Stuck in traffic jam	7
7	Disagreement with workmate	4

Figure 2: Relaxation diary recording attempts to deal with tension

Some people feel diaries over-formalize the process of learning relaxation. However, many people do find them useful and they have a number of functions. In particular, they can be used to monitor progress, and act as a reminder of events that have resulted in tension. Diaries can also identify recurring stressful events that may not have been obvious previously. These are particularly important as their repetitive nature suggests that they may need to be dealt with in some way other than simply trying to relax at the time they occur.

If diaries are used, it is important they become an integral part of the counselling process – a reminder of events to be discussed and learned from. Thus, in the relaxation groups I run, the first part of any session is spent discussing progress during the previous week, using diaries as reminders of key events.

In vivo relaxation. After one or two weeks of monitoring tension and learning relaxation, patients should be encouraged to gradually incorporate relaxation into their daily lives. This can be done by using tension as a cue to attempt to relax, as well as by trying to do so at set intervals, such as in coffee breaks or on the hour. Alternatively, reminders may be built into the environment. One simple strategy is to stick little red dots on a variety of objects in the environment to act as cues to relax. These can be extremely useful if attached to objects which may be triggers to tension such as telephones or watches.

Ideally, relaxation should be used to reduce even relatively low levels of tension. Accumulated stress and gradually increasing tension resulting from a failure to relax when dealing with minor hassles throughout the day can be far more wearing than the occasional big problem which makes us particularly tense. In addition, the constant use of relaxation skills can prepare the person to cope with times of greater stress. Without practice it is difficult to use relaxation skills on such occasions. Equally, relaxation can be used before entering a stressful situation to pre-empt any build up of tension. It is more easy to relax away low, rather than high, levels of tension; the earlier relaxation is used, the better.

The speed and level of relaxation achieved at these times will differ from that gained in relaxation practice (one cannot lie down and practise deep relaxation in a supermarket queue!). However, the goal is the same as that in relaxation practice: systematically attempting to minimize excess tension throughout the muscle groups in the body.

Many people find that initially slowing breathing and taking deep breaths is a good trigger to relaxation. The order in which muscles are relaxed is relatively unimportant, although if they are relaxed in the same order as the relaxation tape this helps maintain the practice in real life. Some people may find they become particularly tense in only certain muscle groups, and they may need initially to concentrate on these.

Continuing relaxation. To be useful, relaxation needs to be integrated into daily life – its use must become a habit. Unfortunately, relaxation cannot be learnt by occasional practice. To be able to relax under the stress of daily hassles, it needs to be a well learned skill. Initially, practice of deep and then quick relaxation needs to be regular (ideally daily, although in practice only a few patients achieve this), and consistent. This should take place over a period of weeks until the patient has mastered the skills of relaxation at times of stress. After this, it may still be useful for patients to listen to the relaxation tape on, say, a weekly or fortnightly basis to remind them how it feels to be fully relaxed, and to avoid slipping back to previous levels of tension without realizing it.

Case Study

Mr J enjoyed the cut and thrust of sales, having turned down promotion to area manager so he could continue direct selling – and incidentally earn more money! Despite a serious MI Mr J continued in his job. However, on two occasions he had been admitted to the CCU following massive episodes of angina, which he had interpreted as a further MI. After the second of these episodes he was seen by a psychologist.

From an initial discussion, it became clear that while he enjoyed the challenge of his job, it involved high levels of stress and tension. Before seeing a potential client he would become 'hyped up', and if he made a big sale he became equally excited and tense. Apart from his work he felt he was not under particular stress, although he reported he liked to be 'on the go' all the time, and he found it hard to relax. As this tension seemed to be contributing to his angina, it was mutually agreed he would learn relaxation. Accordingly, between the first and second appointments, he kept a tension diary in which he noted his average daily tension, and one or two triggers to particularly high levels of tension.

At the second appointment, Mr J reported that he had been able to identify a number of triggers to tension. These included, as expected, occasions at work, in particular either when driving to see clients or when he was with them. More unexpectedly, he also identified that he became quite tense at home when dealing with his two children. He often became irritated and even angry, and these feelings were accompanied by quite high levels of tension. He had never before thought of irritation as stress. However, he was now aware of this state as both emotionally stressful, and also as placing a strain on his heart.

The results of his diary-keeping combined with his previous history reinforced the potential benefits of relaxation to Mr J. About 20 minutes of the next session was used to teach deep relaxation techniques, which he enjoyed. The counsellor recorded the relaxation instructions on an audio-cassette, which Mr J took home and listened to daily. He also continued his tension diary.

The following week, Mr J reported that he had practised relaxation on most days. He also found that as he learned what it felt like to be fully relaxed, he became more aware of times of tension during the day. Indeed, he was now aware of more chronic levels of tension almost continually through his day. He also found he was becoming more relaxed after listening to the tape at home. Initially, he had found it more difficult to relax with the tape than with the counsellor. He had also initially felt somewhat self-conscious when going to the bedroom to practise with the tape. Nevertheless, he felt he was making good progress.

During the next two or three weeks, Mr J continued to practise relaxation using the tape, and began to try to relax when he became aware of increasing tension. He added to his tension diary by recording when he used relaxation techniques during the day, and how successful they had been.

Keeping his diary made Mr J aware of triggers to, or times of, tension, some of which he began to cope with differently. For example, he tried to keep as relaxed as possible while driving to see clients, and tried to space his appointments through the day so he did not have to rush between them. Mr J also got into the habit of putting on the hand brake while stationary in traffic, checking his tension levels and trying to relax. Before seeing clients he would relax for a minute or so while in the car park. He found it relatively easy to relax at these times. More difficult were times when he could not concentrate easily on relaxation, for example, while making a sale, or, in particular, when one of his children was disobedient or annoyed him. On such occasions he either completely forgot to try and reduce any tension, or was unable to concentrate on staying relaxed.

After three weeks of practising deep relaxation, Mr J became a little bored with the tape and felt he was becoming reasonably competent at relaxation. He therefore began to practise quick relaxation on a (nearly) daily basis. Over the next few weeks, two key changes occurred; first, simply through practice, Mr J became more able to relax at times of stress; second, and perhaps more importantly, he reported that he was gradually becoming more relaxed in general. Some things that had previously wound him up no longer did so, not because he was able to deal consciously with any tension, but because he did not become tense in the first place.

One aspect of Mr J's stress, in relation to his angina, required more than relaxation techniques to help. This part of the intervention is described next.

Cognitive Strategies

We all think about and try to explain things which happened to us in the past, or try to think about what may happen in the future. We wonder why a friend did not wave to us in the street; we anticipate a good night out with our friends. It is the explanations we give ourselves about such events and our expectations for the future which affect our mood and behaviour. We do not *know* why our friend did not wave, nor do we *know* we will have a good time out; these are guesses or judgements. They are generally based on previous experience, although our mood at the time can also affect the judgements we make. If we are feeling low, we tend to have less positive expectations for the future and are more likely to attribute pessimistic explanations to events.

The fact that we can make different judgements about things which happen to us or about how we will feel in the future provides the central rationale for cognitive therapy. It assumes that all our thoughts in some way distort or only provide a partial picture of reality. They are hypotheses, a subset of possible explanations.

Most of the time we make fairly accurate judgements or have positive expectations; at other times we tend to see things in a negative light. Emotional problems may arise when we continually view things in a negative light. The core of cognitive therapy is to break the train of negative thoughts, and to modify or replace them with those that are more positive and constructive.

Cognitive strategies and the Egan model

Most stress-related problems are at least associated with stress-engendering thoughts. Thus, if a client identifies stress as one of their problems, part of the initial problem identification phase of the counselling process should attempt to identify any thought processes which are contributing to their stress. Cognitive interventions need not be seen as separate to the Egan model of counselling; they involve the same process of problem identification, goal-setting, and problem resolution as any other aspect of counselling.

Problem identification. Thoughts which add to the stress process can be identified using the investigative techniques of the Egan method (page 39); the only thing to differ is the focus on the thoughts an individual has at times of stress or distress. It is important to identify specific thoughts which occurred in specific situations as this has a number of benefits; it clarifies the link between thoughts and emotions or behaviour, and allows specific solutions to specific problems to be identified. In the example below, Mr S is talking to a helper about events which make him tense, and which may lead to an episode of angina. In this case, the trigger is apparently very trivial. Note the use of empathic feedback, prompting, and direct questioning.

Mr S: *One thing that really gets me uptight is when my daughter makes such a mess in the house . . . well, in her room.*

Helper: *That really annoys you. Can you tell me why?*

Mr S: *I don't know . . . It just winds me up every time it happens. I'm getting angry just thinking about it!*

Helper: *I can see.*

Mr S: *Yes . . . I'm really getting quite uptight just thinking about it.*

Helper: *This seems quite an important source of stress. Can you help me get a better understanding of what happens? Think back to the last time you got angry about the mess your daughter had made. Talk me through what happened. Tell me how you felt, and what you were thinking at the time.*

Mr S: *OK. It was yesterday . . . I got home and went up to get changed. As I went past Jane's room I could see the mess. I just thought to myself, 'This is ridiculous. The girl is 18 years old, and still her room's a mess! Does she think her mother's going to sort it out for her yet again!?' I felt angry and frustrated that she still expects her mother to do all the work for her even at her age.*

Identifying goals. The notion that thoughts affect stress, and that changing thoughts may successfully reduce stress may be new to some people. Because of this, although the problem identification stage may have made the link between thoughts and emotions clear, this may not necessarily immediately lead to these being identified as change goals. A number of strategies may be necessary to facilitate this process. Three may be particularly pertinent: summarizing, challenging, and providing information.

Summarizing is frequently used to provide a link between the problem-identification and goal-identification stages of counselling. It may be particularly useful where a person's thoughts contribute to their problems, as such a link may not have previously been apparent. Summarizing may make these links more explicit, and encourage patients to see such thoughts as potential targets for change:

Helper: *Listening to your description of that particular stressful incident, it seems to me there were a number of things going on. Correct me if I'm wrong or misunderstood something, but it seems that several things happened which resulted in your anger. First, you saw a situation, one I expect with which you were very familiar. As you looked at it some anger-provoking thoughts, such as, 'The girl is 18 years old and still her room's a mess! Does she think her mother's going to sort it out for her yet again!?', came into your head. This, in turn, made you feel tense and angry.*

This summary orients Mr S towards the importance of his thought processes in leading to his anger, yet subtly reflects the framing of his experience in an empathic rather than didactic manner. This may be further developed by discussing other stressful episodes and drawing out the processes involved in each.

Critical to each episode is that the re-conceptualization process is not a didactic presentation or a lecture. Each reframing should be presented as a possible view of events, with frequent checks made on whether the helper's interpretation of events is mirrored by that of the patient. Such phrases as 'Correct me if I'm wrong', 'Have I missed something?', or, 'Is this the way you see it?' engages them in a dialogue in which they are encouraged to view the stress process in a way which will encourage positive change. This approach breaks the stress process down into clearly defined processes, and moves the patient from a view of stress as an incoherent whole which feels impossible to change, into a series of parts, some of which may be amenable to change.

A further way of orientating people to see that thinking differently about a situation may be useful is through the use of challenge; in particular, using challenges as an invitation to explore different ways of looking at problems.

Helper: *Hmmm ... The way you describe that incident shows how your thoughts led to your feeling angry. I wonder whether if you had been able to look at the situation in a different way, whether that may have avoided you feeling this way.*

This type of challenge both tells the patient, implicitly, that there are alternative ways of seeing a situation, as well as inviting them to try and explore these.

If summarizing or challenging do not orientate the patient towards identifying stress-provoking thoughts as a potential area of change, the more explicit provision of information may do so. Here, the helper takes, briefly, a more directive role, in which they explain how thoughts may affect the stress process, and how changing such thoughts may help the patient cope better with their stress. This may be through describing everyday examples or accounts of the successes previous patients have had. In the following dialogue, the helper uses summary as a bridge, before invoking the successes of previous patients as a means of encouraging Mr F to examine his thought processes.

Helper: *Correct me if I'm wrong, but I'm struck by how important your thoughts seem to be in getting you stressed. For example, you feel angry with your workmates because you feel they are making too many demands on you and they are being unfair. You have similar thoughts about your kids. They annoy you because they are too demanding and don't give you time to relax when you get home. One of the important things related to all these incidents is that you get so angry that you feel you don't cope with the situation effectively. Your anger gets in the way.*

Mr F: *Yes. I understand how my thoughts wind me up. But that doesn't get us very far.*

Helper: *Well, it seems to me that if we could somehow find a way to stop your thoughts winding you up in the first place, it may help you keep more calm and deal with the situation more effectively. Many of the people I've seen have tried a number of strategies to help them to do this, and used them very successfully. I wonder if it may be worth exploring some of these to see if they may be useful to you . . .*

Note that, although the helper strongly suggests a way for the sessions to proceed, the final choice of action is left to Mr F.

Changing self-talk

If a goal of changing stress-provoking thought patterns is decided upon, the helper and patient in collaboration can begin to look at ways of altering this internal dialogue. Two major approaches are particularly useful. The first, guided self-dialogue, aims to interrupt the flow of such thoughts by replacing them with more stress-ameliorating ones. The second, cognitive challenge, involves the patient 'capturing' a thought, and trying to rationalize it to a less stress-invoking one. Although the two approaches often merge in practice, here they will be treated separately for clarity.

Guided self-dialogue. At its most basic, guided self-dialogue involves the patient interrupting the flow of negative thoughts – 'I'm never going to manage to cope with my job again'; 'Any minute now', I'm going to feel the pain . . .' – with more positive ones. These typically fall into two broad categories: reminders to use stress coping techniques, and reassuring self-talk.

The first act as reminders to use stress-management skills or coping strategies, such as relaxation, that the patient has already begun to master. Thus, at a time of stress the patient may say to him or herself 'I'm feeling tense – cue relaxation'; or, 'Relax – check out the muscle groups – come on you can do it'; or, 'I'm beginning to get angry – relax . . . slowly'; or, 'You're winding yourself up – calm down, deep breath . . . and relax'; 'Come on – getting het up won't help', and so on.

The second form of self-instruction is more akin to self-reassurance, reminding yourself that you can cope effectively with the feelings or stress at the time. I think of this as giving yourself the reassurance you would want others to give you at a time of difficulty. Thus instructions or statements such as, 'Come on – you've dealt with this before, remember'; 'OK, I had difficulty with this before, but now I can be more successful if I keep calm'; 'This is difficult, but I'm coping – just!', and so on, may help the person keep calm and able to cope with whatever stress they are dealing with.

Once patients begin to understand the link between their thoughts and emotions, they may be encouraged to replace any such stress-inducing thoughts with more appropriate or calming thoughts. Take the example of Mr S (page 66) and the upset he felt about the mess made by his daughter. He could interrupt his anger-invoking thoughts with statements such as:

'Calm down. Getting uptight about this isn't going to help.'
'She doesn't do it to annoy – don't let it wind you up.'
'Come on . . . relax . . . take a deep breath.'
'It's only an untidy room, not the end of the world.'

Imagine a person who becomes angry while waiting in a traffic jam. They may say to themselves:

'Relax . . . Hands off the steering wheel . . . Hand brake on – and relax . . .'
Getting tense isn't going to help – it will only get me flustered and anxious.'
'How relaxed can I get here? Take a deep breath . . . relax . . .'

A third example is of a woman who tends to become angry when dealing with several demands made of her at once. She may make the following statements to help control her irritation or anger:

'Relax. I'm in control. Take a deep breath . . . and relax.'
'Don't take things personally – these people just want the job done.'
'OK, I can't do everything at once. Take it steady and calm. Don't let them get you flustered.'

Note that in each case, the statements combine instructions to use relaxation techniques and statements intended to help rationalize and calm the person's experience of the situation.

To ensure that any dialogue is personally relevant, and to avoid rote repetition which would be of little value, self-talk should be developed by the helper and patient in collaboration, typically through brainstorming techniques and discussion, with prompts where necessary. Such a process involves two steps. First, discussion of what occurred at each time of stress or emotional upset, in particular identifying any thoughts the patient may have had which exacerbated the situation. And second, by discussing any alternative thoughts the patient could have used to defuse it.

It is important that these statements are discussed in the context of particular stressful episodes. That is not to suggest that statements can only be used in situations which have previously been identified and planned. The intention is to teach the patient to both generate and use their own statements at times of stress. Focusing reduces the risk of deriving a banal list of statements, which will be of little value at actual times of stress, such as the ubiquitous, 'Every day, in every way, I'm getting better.' For example:

Helper: *We've identified some of the situations where your self-talk winds you up. Let's look at one of these and think of what you could have said to yourself to help keep you calm.*

Mr D: *OK, I'd like to try and cope when my kids drive me crazy.*

Helper: *That sounds a good one to start with. Think about the last time this happened. What were the thoughts you had that wound you up?*

(Mr D recounts these thoughts.)

Helper: *Can you think of any thoughts that would help you to keep more calm?*

Mr D (pauses): *I guess one thing would be to say to myself, 'Hey, he's only a little guy and he's pleased to see me. I should be thankful, not angry!'*

Helper: *That sounds really good . . .*

(Mr D remains silent.)

Helper: *You've been trying to keep relaxed at times of stress recently. I wonder whether it may be useful to remind yourself to be relaxed. Something like, 'Calm down . . . keep relaxed'?*

Mr D: *That could be useful. I could try that.*

Note that both patient and helper made suggestions of possible statements. If patients have difficulty in generating their own statements, the helper may have to do so. However, any suggestions should be made tentatively, and only after giving a reasonable opportunity for the patient to generate their own.

Once alternative self-statements have been generated, patients may be encouraged to remember them and to use them at times of stress or emotional upset. To help people to remember the statements they have generated, it may be useful to write them down (perhaps with some further suggestions), so they can think them through and rehearse them, or even read the list at times of stress.

Helper: *In our last session, we discussed some of the thoughts and feelings you have in stressful situations and some of the alternative self-statements you might use at such times. I thought it might be useful if I summarized our discussion, so I've written down some statements that you may find useful. I have included your suggestions, and some suggestions other people like yourself have previously found helpful. It may be worth spending a few minutes looking over this list and discussing which you may wish to use at times of stress or emotional upset.*

Cognitive challenge

Cognitive challenge has much in common with guided self-dialogue, as it aims to interrupt the flow of stress-engendering thoughts. However, it differs in one key way: rather than provide a flow of reassuring or instructional thoughts, it encourages the patient to question the *accuracy* of some of their stress-engendering self-talk – to treat stress-engendering thoughts as hypotheses, and to test out the accuracy of each. Mr W (page 54) provides an example of how this can be done. His catastrophizing thoughts were:

'I've got heart disease! Jeez, I'm only 34 . . . that's really bad . . . This must mean I'm really unfit and my health is shot . . . I could have a heart attack at any time! That could be it . . . Am I going to die?'

'Even if I do live, this heart disease is going to mess things up . . . It's not as if me and the boss get on well. I'm going to need time off to recover. That could be it; he won't like that; I could be fired. And what about my social life? I won't have any money. But what would I need that for anyway? I'm hardly going to be going out much any more with the boys . . .'

'Oh, no! My chest hurts again . . . I'm not getting better . . . If I push myself it's going to hurt more . . . I can't do anything right . . . If I exercise it hurts, and that can't be right. If I don't exercise then I'm never going to get better.

Some self-challenges Mr W could make to such thoughts could be:

'This is pretty frightening. But the nurse says that my prognosis is good. If I change a few things (I know I eat too many fatty foods) I can do a lot to help myself. I've just got to put some effort into this . . .

'What evidence do I have that my boss will give me the sack? Well, he doesn't think that badly of me . . . and I've been a good worker. He's usually pretty tolerant . . . I guess he may well help me out. Anyway, my friends won't let me down; they never have in the past. I'm sure they'll be there when I come out . . .'

'*Don't panic! My chest hurt yesterday, but nothing happened, even though I got stressed up about it. If my heart can survive that, it can cope with this now . . . It's probably me worrying and being too conscious of my heart rather than any problem . . .*'

In some ways, Mr W provides a poor example of how cognitive challenge can be used, as his challenges were predominantly based on what he had been told by others. The case of Mr J provides a better example of where the patient's own experiences can be used to help them challenge stress-inducing thoughts. Earlier, I described how relaxation techniques had helped Mr J to cope with some of the stresses involved in his job, and reduced the number of episodes of angina he was having (page 64). However, he did occasionally experience angina, which he now attributed to stress. These episodes were particularly difficult for Mr J to deal with because they awakened memories of his MI and worries about its recurrence. His thoughts ran along the lines of:

'*Oh, no! That pain again. It must be angina! No! It's worse than that . . . It isn't going away! I'm having another heart attack!*'

Because of the panic brought about by these thoughts, Mr J had driven himself, or been driven, to hospital on two occasions and was admitted to CCU with a suspected MI. On both occasions he was found to have had 'only' an episode of angina. Because of his tendency to catastrophize whenever he had angina, he and his helper spent some time working on how he could avoid doing this. Using brainstorming techniques, they explored what strategies he could employ to calm himself down and avoid the feelings of panic he felt at such times. A number of self-dialogue statements and cognitive challenges were thought through in an attempt to help Mr J to use his relaxation techniques and GTN (glycerine trinitrate) tablets to help control his panic and angina. He talked these through within the counselling session:

'*OK. Here's the pain. But you've had this before, and it's only been angina. Take a deep breath and sit down. Relax and take a GTN . . . Concentrate on relaxing . . . chest, arms, stomach. It hurts – but it's different to the heart attack. It feels like angina. It'll go in time. Don't worry. Getting uptight will make it worse. Take a few minutes . . . relax. Yeah, it's getting easier . . . Just keep relaxed, you'll be all right. Come on, they said your heart's in great shape; and you're exercising well. You haven't done anything to cause any problems, so just relax . . .*'

The plan was that Mr J would use these strategies if and when he had any future angina attacks. Sad to say – or perhaps fortunately – the value of these strategies was not put to the test. Mr J did indeed experience further episodes of angina, but did not panic. Talking the issues through, and getting him to challenge and rationalize his fears, even in the relative safety of the counselling session, may have prevented his panic taking him over on future occasions.

Just as relaxation techniques are gradually integrated into the daily routine, so patients can be encouraged to increasingly use their self-talk to help them keep as mentally relaxed as possible, in particular at times of potential stress. Following each session, patients will have a clear goal to achieve in the following week or weeks. This may involve, for example, using self-talk to help minimize feelings of anger at specific instances during the week. Each subsequent session should examine whether the strategies used to help achieve the goal were useful, and if not, why not. Were there unseen problems? If so, goals may be changed or different strategies adopted.

Putting It All Together

So far, cognitive and relaxation methods have been treated as separate and distinct strategies. In practice, most stress-management based interventions try to incorporate them into a coherent whole. Meichenbaum (1985) has developed a model of how such integrated interventions can be developed. It focuses on three questions that people can ask themselves in relation to a stress episode: 'What should I do?'; 'What should I say to myself?'; and, 'How can I stay relaxed?' These issues can be thought through before, during, and, importantly, after a stressful episode.

Rehearsal and coping

Many of the stresses we are likely to encounter, or situations that are likely to lead to feelings of anxiety or depression, are known to us. This knowledge means we can prepare to deal with them, to reduce their adverse impact. We can rehearse our coping responses, for example, while quietly sitting in a chair with plenty of time to think of potential responses to stress. This involves planning three dimensions of the coping response: behaviour, self-talk, and physical tension.

Some plans can be very specific. If a person is expecting a particular problem, they may think about how, specifically, to cope with it. Other plans may be more schematic, and involve thinking about how to deal with more diverse situations, such as how to cope effectively with feelings of anger (see Chapter 5).

The case of Mr J illustrates the strategies he identified in a counselling session to help him cope with feelings of panic during an episode of angina:

What I will do: Make my excuses if I am with anyone and try to get somewhere alone – perhaps try to get to my car.
Sit down, and try to relax.

What I will say to myself: *'OK. Here is the pain. But you've had this before, and it's only been angina. Take a deep breath and sit down. Relax and take a GTN...Concentrate on relaxing ... chest, arms, stomach. It hurts – but it's different to the heart attack. It feels like angina – It'll go in time. Don't worry. Getting uptight will make it worse. Just keep relaxed. You'll be alright.*

Keeping relaxed: Use deep relaxation techniques.
Focus on each muscle, particularly my shoulders and stomach muscles.

Mr S, who you may remember had feelings of panic when he exercised (page 52), may have thought through and utilized the following plan if he had feelings of panic while exercising:

What I will do: Stop exercising, but only for a few minutes while I collect my thoughts.
Sit down if I can for a few moments.
When I feel able, start to exercise again, but very gently.

What I will say to myself: *'Calm down. Most of your feelings are due to panic, not because of your heart.*
Try to relax. Slow your breathing. Don't let it take you over.
OK, I've had these feelings before, and it was a false alarm. This is no different to last time.
I'm not feeling any pain. It's just my heart thumping because of the exercise. Even trained athletes' hearts beat a bit extra when they exercise! It's totally normal'.

Keeping relaxed: Try to keep as relaxed as possible all over.
Remember to take deep slow breaths.
Concentrate on relaxing shoulders, arms, and stomach.

Of course, not all situations can be prepared for in advance. However, the rehearsal stage need not necessarily be prolonged or complex.

Sometimes when events occur there is little time to prepare for coping effectively, and plans may have to be developed on the spot. However, many patients recount how a few seconds' thought may have made quite a difference to how they dealt with a situation, as in the case of Ms E, who was learning stress-management skills to reduce her blood pressure.

Ms E was a cookery demonstrator. Part of her job involved giving demonstrations of cooking in schools. One day, she arrived at a school to be met by an agitated teacher who said that rather than demonstrate to one class, as expected, they wanted her to do two demonstrations, one immediately following the one she had prepared for. Her reaction to this request was to become tense, and to try madly to sort out two demonstrations. This involved a quick trip to the shops, frantically washing up between demonstrations, and giving two rushed demonstrations before frantically driving off to her next appointment.

As Ms E had found the whole incident very stressful, she discussed this at her next counselling session. She examined what her self-talk could have been to help her to keep calm while doing these demonstrations, how she could have tried to keep physically relaxed, and so on. Then she interrupted this flow of thought by saying. 'No, this shouldn't have happened. I became sucked along by the teacher's hassle. If only I had thought for a few seconds I would have realized the impossibility of the situation, and how I was being put upon. I could have refused to do a second demonstration'.

A few seconds' thought would have changed Ms E's response to the stress trigger completely.

Once rehearsal, or preparation to deal with a stressor, has been thought through, the next phase of the coping process is to put these plans into action. This may be more or less successful. For either outcome, some time would usefully be spent in analysing why it was so.

Reflection

I often hear the saying, 'We all learn with experience'. Sadly, this may be true for some people, but by no means all. There is great value in looking back on times of stress and reviewing how they were dealt with as a way of identifying each person's most effective stress-management strategies. Strategies which work can be noted for further use, while those which are not successful can be rejected, to be substituted with alternatives.

Such reflection is probably the least emphasized aspect of stress management training – yet it can be the most powerful aid to managing stress successfully. It encourages people to experiment and to try out different strategies to see which ones suit them best, and not to be downhearted if these are unsuccessful; rather to see them as learning experiences. This takes us back to the fundamental approach of this book: it is the *person* who should be central to the process of stress management, *not the techniques*. While stress management often involves teaching people new skills and ways of coping with stress, it must not be forgotten that the heart of the intervention lies in helping *them* to cope with their problems. They can best determine which skills are most appropriate for them to use, and when to use them.

The goal of counselling is for people to learn to use the rehearsal and reflection stages as a routine way of coping with their problems. These also provide a good model of the counselling process itself: rehearsal is typically conducted through interaction between the helper and patient within a session; the patient then tries to put any plans into action; followed by a form of debriefing in following sessions, which attempts to identify the strengths and weaknesses of any strategies used, and finally, to learn from these to develop better ones.

Summary

❑ If events are seen as threatening and the person feels they will have difficulty coping with them; stressful emotions, behaviours, and physiological states will arise.

❑ Learning stress management may be useful for patients who have obvious stresses in their lives; have stress related angina; or are involved in a preventive or rehabilitation programme to reduce risk of further MI, or where stress is interfering with a patient's rehabilitation.

❑ Relaxation involves three interacting phases: learning relaxation using a relaxation tape; learning to monitor and identify tension in daily life; and learning to use relaxation skills at times of stress.

❑ Two different cognitive strategies are identified: guided self-dialogue, which involves providing reassuring self-talk or reminders to use other coping strategies; and cognitive challenge which involves disputation of stress-engendering thoughts.

❑ Both these, and other, strategies may be brought together through focusing on: rehearsal; coping; and reflection.

5

Risk Factor Intervention

Smoking, low levels of exercise, and Type A Behaviours (TAB) increase risk of heart disease or disease progression. Accordingly, people found to have these risk factors are often advised to modify their behaviour in some way, following either preventive screening, or in the course of a rehabilitation programme.

This advice, however well meant, may be difficult to put into practice. For example, many smokers are aware of the health risks involved in smoking and have tried to give up in the past – and failed. Advice does not always lead to appropriate behavioural change. Many people may not feel the need to change, or may lack the necessary skills or motivation to achieve it should they wish to.

This chapter introduces a number of techniques shown to help people modify behaviours which put them at risk for CHD or disease progression. It focuses on smoking cessation, exercise, and TAB in the context of the approach adopted in the previous chapters, being person-centred and problem-solving.

Thus, although a number of methods of behavioural change are suggested, these should not be seen as prescriptive. While many people have found them helpful, they remain potential solutions to problems which may or may not be relevant to everyone. Some people may already have a good idea of how to set about changing their behaviour: a smoker who has successfully stopped in the past may well have some ideas about the best way of stopping now. People know their own strengths and weaknesses, and what may work best for them. Utilizing these resources, rather than the inappropriate application of standardized techniques, is the key to successful behavioural change.

Counselling Smokers

To understand the difficulties some people have in stopping smoking, it may be helpful to examine *why* people smoke.

To an established smoker, smoking is both a habit and a powerful psychological tool. The nicotine in cigarettes has powerful mood altering properties; it can both increase alertness and concentration, or help to relax and calm the smoker. In addition, nicotine is addictive, and stopping smoking may result in withdrawal symptoms varying from minor lightheadedness and poor concentration to severe symptoms including pounding headaches, dizziness and shaking. A third maintaining factor is that smoking often becomes associated with a number of situations in which a person has smoked, for example, many smokers automatically have a cigarette when they answer the telephone or after a meal, simply out of habit.

Thus, people who stop smoking have three particular problems to cope with: the loss of a powerful psychological support; changing a well-established habit; and the possible onset of unpleasant withdrawal symptoms. Each may pose a formidable hurdle – together they often pose an almost insurmountable barrier. To be effective in helping people give up smoking, account must be taken of each of these elements.

The focus of counselling sessions needs to be the identification and reduction of each of the potential difficulties associated with giving up, which fits well into the third stage of the Egan model. Progress more or less involves setting a series of subgoals (for example, 'Cut down to 15 cigarettes a day'; 'Stop smoking on a predetermined day') in an attempt to achieve the overall goal of cessation. A number of clinicians have identified a series of stages through which many smoking cessation interventions pass, and strategies by which some of the problems identified may be ameliorated; these phases will be discussed later.

While advising someone of the mechanics of stopping smoking can be achieved in one session, more useful would be extended contact with a person over a period of weeks as they cut down, and in the immediate weeks after stopping. Although it is impossible to state how long such counselling should last, the following time-frame may be useful to bear in mind:

Stage 1: Thinking about giving up (initial meeting).
Stage 2: Planning to give up (begins in the first or second meeting, depending on time limitations and how long Stage 1 lasts).
Stage 3: Starting to give up – the smoker gradually cutting down the number of cigarettes smoked (may typically last about two to three weeks).
Stage 4: The 'Stop Day' and beyond – supporting the person through the first few weeks of being a non-smoker (may involve a further three or four meetings at, say, weekly intervals).

Stage 5: Preparing the person for any problems they may face in the longer-term future.

Many established programmes provide group counselling sessions. The reasons for this are both economic and therapeutic. Economically, individual counselling of smokers is expensive and time consuming; therapeutically, many smokers benefit from the motivation provided by a group and enjoy the social aspects involved. However, many people do not want to join groups, and programmes that do not engage in individual counselling miss many opportunities to help people stop. In addition, many people obtain equal, if not greater support, from family, friends and others than they do from group members. The phases of intervention and issues raised within them are similar for both groups and individuals.

Stage 1: Thinking about giving up

About 30 percent of people attending screening clinics smoke cigarettes regularly. Many will have tried to give up at least once in the previous year, and failed, and few will be actively considering stopping smoking. Even amongst people with heart disease, successful cessation rates are not high. The reasons for this are not clear. Some smokers remain unconvinced of the benefits of stopping. Others may see the health benefits of giving up smoking, but may not have sufficient motivation to engage in what they may see as a difficult, or even impossible, task.

Clearly, at this stage, these people would not benefit from immediate discussion about how to give up; this could actually reduce their motivation still further. Rather, the goal of counselling should be to increase their motivation or confidence, and move them to consider the possibility of cessation. This may also be a useful preparation for people who are already committed to giving up smoking, as it may help maintain their motivation if they encounter any difficulties.

Increasing motivation to stop can best be achieved through discussion and brainstorming techniques in which smokers are asked to consider the costs and benefits of giving up. Such techniques allow the helper to help them identify their reasons for wanting to stop smoking. They will also allow the patient to provide information where necessary and to identify and challenge any misconceptions identified. Finally, they forewarn both helper and smoker of possible future problems should they decide to stop smoking.

Exploration of issues should be specific and focused. Discussion of 'average' or 'typical' health benefits of cessation is too impersonal and easily discounted. The discussion should focus on the benefits to the *individual* involved. In particular, thinking through the *immediate* benefits of stopping, such as reducing the risk of angina or being less 'out of puff', may be a more powerful motivator than consideration of longer-term, probabilistic, benefits. (It may be worth encouraging patients to write down some of these benefits, which can be used as a reminder of their reasons for wanting to stop if they have difficulties later.)

Only when a patient has made a clear commitment to attempt to stop smoking, can discussion of how best to achieve this goal begin. It is possible that some people will have strong views about how this can best be accomplished and what sort of help they require. These wishes should be respected wherever practicable and possible. If they request such techniques as hypnosis or acupuncture, any lack of expertise should be admitted. However, it should also be stated that the techniques you may suggest may be equally, if not more, useful in helping them to stop smoking.

The process of quitting typically follows four stages:

- planning to give up;
- cutting down;
- stopping;
- staying stopped.

Negotiation through each stage involves setting a series of goals, and planning how each may best be achieved. Issues and tactics related to each phase will be discussed below. An explanation, and rationale, for the overall plan that may be useful to patients can be found in Appendix C.

Stage 2: Planning to give up

Effective intervention in smoking requires a good understanding of the problem, which allows the patient and helper to develop an intervention that will address the needs of the individual, allowing appropriate problem-solving strategies to be applied. This can be developed during counselling sessions, with patients being asked to think through a typical day and trying to identify when they smoked each cigarette and what triggered it. This approach is useful as it shows the link between smoking and environmental and emotional triggers, of which the smoker may not have previously been aware. This renders smoking more understandable – and hence controllable – than some patients may have previously thought.

Patients may forget instances of smoking, or not notice regularities to the triggers which cue their smoking. To get round this, it may be useful if patients keep a record of when and why they smoke, and how difficult it would be to give up each cigarette smoked. This is best done using a small diary, which can be carried around in, or attached to, cigarette packets.

A diary helps smokers to identify habit cigarettes and what triggers them (coffee breaks, finishing a job around the house, going to the pub, the telephone ringing) and so on). It will also help them to identify how many cigarettes are smoked because of a craving for nicotine. Finally, it will give them some idea as to which cigarettes they may miss out first as they cut down on their smoking. Unless they wish to give up immediately, it may be useful for a patient to keep a diary for a week or so before beginning to give up.

Time	Ease of quitting (0–10)	Trigger
08.00	2	Desperate for a fag! First of the day.
08.05	8	Habit – just enjoy a second.
08.45	6	Driving to work.
10.00	3	Fag break.
10.15	7	With cup of coffee.

Figure 3: Example of smoker's diary

As patients become aware of the triggers to their smoking, they can begin to think of strategies to help them cope with missing out each cigarette they smoke. Although they have not begun to cut down, this will provide some preparation for the next phase of the intervention.

Stage 3: Beginning to give up

There are two obvious ways of stopping smoking. The first, apparently painless, method may be to cut down gradually until the smoker simply smokes so few cigarettes a day that giving up is easy. With the second, they may stop immediately. The patient may have some ideas about which of these two options they would prefer, which should be respected and followed through with the maximum support.

If, however, they are not sure which they would prefer, the best approach may involve a compromise between the two – to cut down smoking over a preliminary period of, say, one or two weeks, to a level of about 12 cigarettes per day, and then to stop completely. Smoking only 12 cigarettes a day is usually sufficient to prevent nicotine withdrawal symptoms, and allows the patient to develop and practise their strategies for dealing with not smoking without the extra strain of dealing with these symptoms. Once smoking levels dip below this, extending the period of cutting down only prolongs these symptoms and increases the risk of the person failing to stop smoking.

If this method is chosen, a number of strategies may be used to achieve the goals set during the cutting-down phase:

* identifying a Stop Day;
* structured reduction;
* trigger avoidance;
* coping with triggers;
* rewarding progress;
* gaining social support.

A logical way of cutting down is to work toward a Stop Day, when the person will attempt to stop smoking completely. By this time a reasonable smoking level would be 12 cigarettes a day. The individual should decide the time period in which they wish to cut down to this level, and work out a gradual reduction of the number of cigarettes smoked each day during this run-down period. They may find it easier to cut out the easier cigarettes before the more difficult. The diary will identify which cigarettes can most easily be missed.

The next task is to identify how the patient may best cope when they feel the urge to smoke, but want to 'cut that one out'. Solutions are best derived through discussion and brainstorming; perhaps focusing on particular cigarettes identified in the smoking diary. While, as always, patients should be encouraged to work through their own solutions, two tried and tested methods may also be used: trigger avoidance, and coping with triggers.

Habit cigarettes are associated with routine events. One approach to cutting down is to avoid or change such situations, as these may trigger a strong desire to smoke, for example, by sitting in a different part of the work canteen or with non-smokers, going for a walk at breaks, or going to no-smoking areas in buses and cinemas. The diary should show frequent triggers to smoking, and brainstorming is effective in thinking of ways of changing or avoiding these triggers to make them less potent:

Helper: *You said earlier that you found it particularly difficult not to smoke when other people were smoking near you. I wonder if we should look at some of these occasions and think how you could make it easier not to smoke* . . .

As in any counselling, if open invitations to work through solutions do not meet with success, more direct prompts may be useful:

Helper: *I wonder whether there are other ways you could spend your break, or perhaps other people you could sit by, until you feel able to resist the urge to smoke when you sit next to smokers during your lunch break* . . .

Of course, it is often impossible, or undesirable, to avoid triggers. Thus, an issue that may usefully be explored is how best to cope with them. One basic but important skill is simply being able to say, 'No, thank you. I don't smoke'. It may sound silly, but many patients find it useful to simply stand in front of a mirror and rehearse saying just that. Distraction is a second approach that may be useful, for example, listening carefully to conversations or trying to keep relaxed. Again, brainstorming may identify a range of tactics that can be used:

Helper: *Looking at your diary, a frequent trigger to your smoking is answering the telephone. I wonder whether there are any ways that you could make it easier not to smoke at this time* . . .

Two other more general issues may usefully be discussed at this stage. Encouraging patients to reward themselves for their successes can be an important boost while they are cutting down and during the first few days or even weeks after quitting. These may be small, for example, watching a favourite video at the end of a successful day; or large, for example going out for a meal at the end of a week. Of course, one important reward is simply pride in the achievement of giving up.

Support from friends is also a key factor in successful quitting. This may well be raised during brainstorming tactics for giving up. If so, it should be encouraged by the helper. If not, the idea may usefully be suggested: 'Have you thought of getting some help from other people while you try to stop?'

Some people may simply wish to tell their friends they are trying to stop and ask for their support. More ambitious patients may wish to stop at the same time as a friend, or even to form a small self-help group. This social support can be an important factor in the success or failure of any attempt to quit.

Nicotine substitutes. Nicotine substitutes have been shown to be of benefit to smokers who are dependent on nicotine, but to be of less use for those whose smoking is largely habitual. A simple rule of thumb to determine dependence on nicotine, is the importance of the first cigarette of the day. If someone feels this would be the most difficult cigarette to give up, they would almost certainly benefit from nicotine substitutes. A look at the diary may provide some further clues. If many cigarettes are smoked because the patient is 'desperate for a cigarette', this may also indicate a high nicotine dependency. Some people may wish to use nicotine substitutes regardless of these academic arguments, and their wishes should be respected.

Nicotine substitutes need not be used regularly until after stopping smoking. However, if they intend to use them, many smokers find it useful to chew some nicotine gum as they begin to miss out cigarettes.

Stage 4: 'Stop Day' and beyond

At some stage, the decision to stop will have to be made by the patient. Once this day is reached, some problems already encountered may continue, while others, notably the onset of withdrawal symptoms, may begin. Continued success depends on utilizing the techniques the person has already found useful, and perhaps trying some further tactics.

Most smokers choose not to smoke at all on their Stop Day; it helps to start a new day with a new habit. Alternatively, a ritual burning of the last remaining cigarettes may help to instil a feeling of positive change.

Coping with craving. About half of those who stop smoking experience strong cravings for a cigarette. These may occur for as long as two or three weeks after stopping, although the first two or three days after quitting are the worst. The urge to smoke typically comes in short spells, each peak lasting two or three minutes with periods of relative ease in between. As time goes on, the craving becomes less severe and at longer intervals. One simple strategy that patients may find helpful at this time is to simply keep busy, so that there is no time to be bored and to think of smoking. Other strategies can again be identified through brainstorming.

It is important to try to generate a positive outlook towards these and other withdrawal symptoms, which may include sweating, tremors, and fatigue. They can be reframed to be seen as 'signs of recovery'; as an indication of the body getting rid of nicotine. Each craving represents one step further along the road to fitness and abstinence. If withdrawal effects are severe, this is an indication that the patient would benefit from the use of a nicotine substitute.

Avoiding and coping with triggers. If the smoker has used a smoking diary, they should be well aware at this stage of any high-risk situations, when they are likely to be highly tempted to smoke. In the first few days after stopping, when temptation is at its greatest, patients may find it easiest to avoid such triggers when possible, gradually coming into contact with them as their confidence grows. Otherwise, coping strategies practised in the cutting down phase will have to be used to their full. Some people feel they have to carry a packet of cigarettes with them at this time 'just in case'. However, I try to challenge this notion as its seems to be putting temptation rather too close.

'If I should slip . . .'. Many people smoke at least one cigarette after their Stop Day. It is important that this does not become a catastrophe, and they continue to smoke, because they have 'already failed'. It may, therefore, be useful to discuss an emergency drill which patients can use if they give in to temptation. Some find it useful to write it down on a bit of card which they carry with them, so they can re-motivate themselves if necessary. It goes along the following lines:

'To err is human. To have one cigarette does not mean that all my hard work has been in vain, or that I have no will power. It does not mean that I have to continue smoking.'

'Stop smoking now! Not tomorrow. Not next week. Avoid the cop-out response of, 'Since I smoked today I might as well go ahead and smoke as much as I want and stop smoking tomorrow'. There is always the danger that tomorrow never comes.'

To maintain motivation it may help to have on the same card two of the key reasons why the patient wants to stop smoking. These may act as a further prompt to control.

Nicotine replacements after Stop Day. Nicotine substitutes can be obtained in 2mg and 4mg strengths. Most smokers need only use the 2mg strength, with only a small minority needing the higher nicotine level. Initially, patients electing to use nicotine replacements can use them regularly (within the recommended limits) through the day. However, it is important to begin cutting down on their use as soon as patients feel able. Some studies report people still use them as long as one year after stopping smoking, and patients may need to be encouraged to cut down and avoid a long-term dependence on these drugs. Just as patients may establish targets to cut down the number of cigarettes they smoke, these may also be useful in reducing their use of nicotine substitutes.

Stage 5: Staying stopped

Many smokers succeed in giving up smoking for days, weeks, or even months – and then begin to smoke again. For this reason, towards the end of the counselling period it is extremely important to prepare them to cope with any future temptation. Appropriate counselling should have begun to teach the patient problem-solving skills, which may help them to deal with temptations in the future. Nevertheless, patients may usefully be advised to:

- Avoid complacency. One of the commonest reasons for starting to smoke again is that people simply 'felt like having a cigarette', or had 'just one or two' and became hooked on smoking again. These danger signs should be identified and avoided.
- Take care in situations previously identified as high risk, particularly smoking while drinking. Alcohol is a well-known destroyer of good resolutions.
- Be assertive if offered a cigarette; for example, saying, 'No, thank you. I don't smoke' is more powerful and positive than, 'No, thank you. I've given up'.
- Be prepared to cope with craving. Some ex-smokers report occasional strong urges to smoke long after any withdrawal period. These do not last very long, but patients need to be forewarned.

Some final considerations. How much time should be spent with a person while they give up smoking? This must be a compromise between the time and commitment available from the helper and the needs of the patient. For some patients, one meeting may suffice; for others a series of meetings lasting, say, half an hour each, may be necessary.

To optimize the effectiveness of these meetings, it is important that at the end of each meeting an informal contract is made in which the patient agrees to attempt to achieve a behavioural goal; 'Cut down to 12 a day'; 'Stop on the day of the next meeting'. If this goal is not achieved, then the goals need to be revised or the meetings stopped. Such agreements provide a clear measure of progress, and indicate whether there remains any value to their continuing.

Finally, it may be worth being available at the end of a telephone for five minutes each day so that patients can contact the helper for a brief chat should they need it. In some cases this may be the most valuable few minutes of the entire intervention.

Improving Fitness

It is not possible for this book to deal adequately with all aspects of exercise in relation to heart disease. Most are better dealt with by exercise physiologists or physiotherapists. However, psychologists have been particularly active in research and intervention into two key, related, aspects of exercise: motivation to exercise, and improving adherence to exercise regimes. Here, both will be discussed in relation to rehabilitation programmes, although the issues discussed are of relevance to anyone advising patients to begin a programme of exercise.

While the majority of people enjoy taking part in exercise rehabilitation programmes, only a minority continue to exercise afterwards. This is disappointing, because the maximal benefits can only come from sustained and regular exercise. For a programme to be effective, it needs not only to encourage attendance and exercise between meetings, but to encourage attenders to continue exercising in the future. Of course, some people simply do not want to take up exercise – they never have, and they never will, and their wishes should be respected. However, many who may think about doing so, also fail to take up longer-term exercise, despite enjoying it in the rehabilitation setting.

A number of issues likely to affect participation in, or continued exercise following, rehabilitation programmes are discussed below. The section is divided into programme design issues – dealing with aspects of designing or running exercise programmes – and generalization issues – factors designed to encourage exercise beyond the confines of the rehabilitation gym.

Programme design issues

Rationalizing perceived risks. Exercise rehabilitation programmes often prove paradoxical to patients: while they can see some logic in them, many feel some disquiet when asked to engage in exercise which they understand stresses the heart, and may result in angina or a further heart attack. This understandably makes some patients reluctant to engage in exercise, particularly beyond the safety of a well-staffed and equipped gym.

It is important that any programme is sensitive to these issues and helps to minimize, or rationalize, such anxiety. This can be achieved explicitly by explanation of the processes involved in exercise, and, implicitly, by organizing them to maximize perceptions of safety. For example, patients who have undergone exercise programmes where their cardiac state is initially monitored using ambulatory ECGs report feeling able to exercise more rigorously because of the feelings of safety this brings. This level of monitoring is, unfortunately, rare and expensive. Regular monitoring of heart rate allows rather less sophisticated reassurance that the person will not be allowed to over-exert themselves within sessions.

Perhaps more important is to prevent such anxieties occurring between sessions. Patients may be encouraged to exercise by learning to recognize what a safe and unsafe degree of exercise feels like, which may be given through treadmill tests, where patients are given feed-back at different degrees of effort about what is safe or unsafe for them.

The influence and concerns of partners must also be considered. Many have an understandable fear of patients over-exerting them-selves, and may even try to dissuade them from engaging in what they think of as 'too much exercise'. One way that such concerns may be allayed is to involve the partner in the exercise programme. For example, those who are present at treadmill testing – and who are therefore shown how much exercise is safe – feel much less anxious about their partner exercising, and are more likely to encourage them to do so, than those who are not given such information.

Goal-planning. There have been many attempts to identify the optimum level of exercise that should be incorporated into an exercise programme. Some studies have found better adherence to pro-grammes which involve quite low levels of exercise; others have found increased adherence to programmes which involve higher levels.

If the level of exercise likely to encourage people to exercise beyond the programme differs, it does so in a consistent way: people are most likely to continue exercising if the level of exercise in a programme is sufficiently demanding to give them some satisfaction from taking part and makes them feel 'fitter', but is not so demanding that it leaves them exhausted and tired. Worst of all, is if the level of exercise is such that it makes them anxious that they are 'overdoing things'. This argues strongly for the development of individualized exercise programmes.

A graded increase towards a desirable target level may provide a powerful incentive to exercise. As ever, goals should be established through a negotiation process, not set by an 'expert'. Care must be taken to ensure that the goals are achievable, but sufficiently demanding that the patient feels they are making tangible progress.

Some people benefit from keeping an exercise diary to plan their goals, either in the rehabilitation gym or beyond. Weekly or daily targets such as 'Walk briskly for 20 minutes three times this week'; or, 'Jog for 20 minutes without a rest', can be planned, and times identified when they will be carried out. This may help to prioritize exercise. Putting a commitment down on paper seems to make it more concrete, and can prevent other things getting in the way.

Diaries can also be used to record progress, such as how far a walk was or for how long it lasted. They can be made rather more interesting by recording other information, such as how a run went or felt, who the person ran with, and so on. Over time, a diary can give encouragement, by allowing people to monitor their progress, and by reminding them of the more pleasurable aspects of exercise.

Generalization issues

A primary goal of any rehabilitation programme should be to encourage participants to maintain some degree of exercise after discharge. As patients will almost inevitably run into some difficulties, it may be worth trying to pre-empt some of these through discussions, in which potential future problems are identified and solutions thought through. Boredom, isolation, and time problems may all militate against exercise. Some ways of minimizing these potential problems are discussed below.

Minimizing boredom. At the beginning of any exercise programme boredom is unlikely to be an issue. Only later, when periods of exercise are longer and less novel, is it likely to become a problem. The ideal way to avoid boredom is to engage in a form of exercise which is intrinsically interesting. Unfortunately, this may not always be possible, at least in the early days.

While more rigorous exercise may be a later goal, many people initially both need and prefer to engage in exercise which is less stressful and more controllable. For this reason, many people take up walking or jogging, which has many advantages: it develops aerobic fitness; it does not require much equipment or time and effort spent in booking facilities or finding partners; and perhaps most importantly, it is eminently controllable – if you want to stop, you do so. However, its major drawback is that it can be quite boring.

There are no particular methods of providing instant relief from boredom, although there are many approaches that could be tried out. These vary from jogging with a personal radio or cassette (playing quietly to avoid drowning out important noises, such as traffic), to imagining 'movies' in your head. If jogging alone, diverse and interesting routes can be found, although, however pleasant, familiar jogging routes may become boring. Most of us take in very little of our surroundings when we exercise. But they are constantly changing and developing: the experience of running through a park may differ on each occasion and from season to season. Concentrating on one's surroundings and how they change can alter the interest of a run quite markedly. Other techniques may involve distraction, such as counting the number of fellow joggers seen and waved to; or thinking about all the food to be eaten at the end (another favourite).

Social aspects. Exercising in company is probably one of the most powerful influences in maintaining exercise. Despite the disadvantages of requiring time and effort to organize, it has enormous benefits. As well as the enjoyment of sharing an activity with someone else, exercising with others may help allay any anxiety about having a further MI without help being at hand. Exercising in company also has a motivational aspect: after arranging to meet a friend at a certain time and place, it is difficult to opt out and not exercise. In the context of group exercise rehabilitation, the leader of the group may usefully facilitate the development of a buddy network of those who would like to exercise together during the programme, or after they have left it.

Coping with time problems. It is often difficult to fit programmed exercise into a busy daily schedule, particularly where this has not been a previous priority. One way to maintain an exercise regime in the face of conflicting demands is to set aside time to exercise at regular intervals, and to ensure these times are not seen to be expendable. If time is not set aside, exercise is frequently replaced by other activities, and the habit is either not established or lost. Of course, some changes to daily routine may have to be negotiated with family members, but most are only too happy to accept changes that may prevent disease progression.

An alternative way to maintain or increase levels of exercise is to make it an integral part of daily living. Simple changes to daily life can ensure fitness without engaging in potentially disruptive levels of exercise. These involve maximizing everyday opportunities to engage in relatively low levels of exercise, such as brisk walking.

The cumulative effect of making the most of such opportunities is frequently sufficient to promote cardiovascular fitness. For example, if work is not far, it may be possible to walk briskly from home. If it is further, then an alternative strategy may be to get off the bus or train or park the car some distance from work and walk to and from this point. This technique may be applied equally when going shopping, popping out to the newsagent, visiting friends, and so on.

Type A Behaviour

Many people, whether they have heart disease or not, think that stress plays a major role in the development of CHD, and frequently seek some advice about how to reduce it. Some methods have already been examined (Chapter 4). These techniques have so far been applied to situations in which stress has been seen as stemming from environmental factors or problems in coping with rehabilitation. In addition, some programmes have attempted to help people change a style of behaviour which directly puts them at increased risk of heart disease or re-infarction.

The archetypal Type A person is someone who is always on the go, quick to anger, and who tries to fit more and more into less and less time. Type As characteristically talk quickly, are prone to interrupt others, but do not allow themselves to be interrupted. They frequently report doing more than one thing at a time, tend to rush things, and do not like being held up. They are also prone to frequent angry feelings and behaviours, an attribute thought to be most closely associated to CHD.

There are a number of formal assessments of TAB. However, my favourite, although not infallible, diagnostic criterion was recounted to me by a coronary care charge nurse. He said that he could always tell which patients were Type A, even without talking to them. They were the people, who, when given a bowl of water and advised to wash themselves carefully, ignored all such cautionary advice and were soon rigorously washing themselves and spilling water all over their bed. I am yet to be convinced of the diagnostic accuracy of this particular assessment, but it serves to give a sense of the vigour of these people. Mr D was one of the more extreme Type A men who attended a stress-management course as part of a primary care-based intervention to reduce his high blood pressure.

Case Study

Mr D, a travelling salesman, was an imposing man being six feet tall and seeming six feet wide. Unlike most salesmen who have to make repeat visits to clients, the commodity Mr D sold involved one-off negotiations. Accordingly, he did not have to build good client relations, and his sales tactics were intimidatory rather than conciliatory. If the 'punter' refused to buy his product, he would put the price up and edge closer to them. These tactics were successful: he was the firm's number one salesman, earned a small fortune, and had won many prizes for his sales. In fact, he attended the stress management course following a free trip to the Bahamas.

Mr D's day would follow a typical pattern. He made appointments on the hour for all his meetings. In order to achieve this timing – he had to travel between clients – he had to execute short bursts of rapid driving (he was fined for speeding two weeks into the group), during which time he became aggressive and argumentative with fellow drivers. He told the group he had pushed two cars off the road to get them out of his way when he had been in a particular hurry!

Mr D worked long hours, but away from work pushed himself just as hard. He played squash competitively and hated to lose. He even competed in how much beer he could drink in the evening at the pub! When it was suggested that some of these behaviours may have been contributing to his raised blood pressure Mr D was extremely sceptical. Indeed, he felt that he enjoyed life and had everything to lose if he changed his behaviour. Nevertheless, he did attend the stress-management group, (of which more later).

People may begin to think about changing their behaviour as a result of various influences. Some may recognize their behaviour as being stressful and actively seek help in reducing this source of stress. Some may become aware through counselling that some Type A characteristics, such as feeling angry or hostile, are causing them problems, either because they are triggering angina attacks or causing them personal difficulties. Other people may become involved in trying to change their behaviour as part of a risk-education programme (Chapter 6).

The initial approach taken with people coming from these differing starting points may vary. Nevertheless, each person comes with a goal of changing some aspect of their behaviour. The actual behaviour to be changed, and the means by which this can best be done, involves the typical sequence of counselling events: goal-setting, identifying how these goals can be achieved, and working through any problems which arise while trying to achieve them.

TAB modification falls into the Egan model of counselling, and all its techniques are applicable here. The next section will identify some techniques which may be useful in helping people to change their behaviour. These are explored in more detail by Roskies (1988).

Helping people to change Type A behaviours essentially employs the same strategies as helping them cope with more general stresses. However, the goal of change becomes more specific: to alter their responses to environmental triggers to a less aggressive and pressured style.

Monitoring behaviour

Unlike general stress management training, where behavioural change may not always be a central goal for any intervention, Type A modification does have this as a clear goal. Its aim is to help people identify when they are using Type A behaviours, and to identify and use strategies to change. These goals may be, for example, to reduce the amount they rush, to lessen their aggression or hostility, or to increase the amount of time they spend in a relaxed state.

The first stage of behavioural change involves people identifying when they are engaging in TAB. Some occasions may be obvious, for example when they become irritated or angry, but others may be less so. Most people respond to events around them in a characteristic manner. Because this is typical of them and a style of coping they have lived with for many years, it has become habitual, that is, it is automatic and operates at a low level of awareness. They may not *feel* particularly rushed or aggressive, although neutral observers may see them this way.

The first stage of any intervention, therefore, is to focus patients' attention on when and how they behave in a pressured or aggressive manner, and to identify what triggers such reactions. In counselling terms, this can be seen as problem exploration. This involves some explanation of the types of behaviour which may be considered 'self-stressing', and exploration of these behaviours through discussion and possibly through the use of a diary. This can be used on a daily basis to identify triggers and typical responses to them, allowing the identification of potential future intervention points. A more sophisticated diary may also examine cognitive triggers to TAB, or the degree of physical tension associated with any particular trigger (see Figure 4).

MONDAY

Time	Trigger	Behaviour	Thoughts
07.30	Breakfast	Rushed! Argumentative.	I've got a lot to do today. I'm going to be late!
08.00	Driving to work	Driving fast. Breaking the speed limit. Impatient if held up.	Come on! You may have all day ... I haven't!
11.00	Meeting at work	Irritated by the time it takes to get anything done.	This is ridiculous. We go round and round and never make a decision. What a bloody waste of time!

Figure 4: A typical diary of Type A behaviour

Coping with triggers

Once triggers and their responses have been identified, strategies to change can be developed.

Relaxation. Before tackling Type A behaviours directly, some basic grounding in relaxation techniques can be useful. This may modify behaviour in itself. For example, in discussing the benefits of slowing down his pace of life, one person volunteered that he had already done so: 'If I hadn't, I'd have had whiplash injuries to my neck! It's impossible to rush and be relaxed at the same time ...' Relaxation diaries may be used to help patients become more aware of their TAB and its triggers. Relaxation can be used whenever a person feels rushed or angry. Patients can also be encouraged to become relaxed at times of tension, whether this accompanies TAB or not.

Cognitive techniques. It has been suggested that people who are Type A have a number of characteristic beliefs which underpin their behaviour. For example, they may be less driven by the desire for success than by the fear of failure, which they believe will result in people thinking less of them. The case of Mr P shows how this concern may affect their daily lives.

Mr P, a junior manager for a large construction firm, had driven about 100 miles to a site meeting and thought he was going to be late. Accordingly, he had driven far beyond the speed limit to try to be on time:

Helper: *So you thought you were going to be late. How did you feel about that?*

Mr P: *Typical me, really. I didn't want to be late, so I got uptight and began to drive hard.*

Helper: *How late did you think you were going to be?*

Mr P: *I don't know . . . About ten minutes or so, I would guess.*

Helper: *Why was it so important to be exactly on time?*

Mr P: *I don't really know . . . It's just me I suppose . . . Well, one thing is that I don't want to be the last at the meeting, because it looks bad. It looks like I'm incompetent, and I want people to think I'm doing a good job.*

Two things are of note in Mr P's explanation. His behaviour resulted from anxieties about looking a fool and not the competent person he would like to think himself; and, what is not clear from the vignette is why he was late. Typically, Mr P had set off at the last minute because he was trying to cram too much into his day, with the consequence of almost inevitably being late. One way for Mr P to avoid his anxieties would have been to set off a little earlier, in order to pre-empt the trigger to stress in the first place. But need he have been so concerned when he was in this situation? He and the helper discussed it further:

Helper: *Were you the last at the meeting?*

Mr P: (smiles) *I have to admit, I wasn't. In fact, it started late because some of the other people coming were caught up in traffic.*

Helper: *How did you feel about that?.*

Mr P: *Relieved really. I was glad I didn't hold things up.*

Helper: *How did you feel about the other people being late?*

Mr P: *I was glad they got me out of a spot. But I didn't mind them being late. They were caught up in traffic and couldn't help it. These things happen.*

Helper: *So, you don't think any less of them for being late, or think of them as incompetent. I wonder why you judge yourself more harshly?*

Mr P: *Hmm . . . I do tend to be hard on myself. Perhaps too hard . . .*

Here the helper is beginning to challenge some of the assumptions underlying Mr P's aggressive and time-urgent behaviour. As in more general stress management training, guided self-dialogue and cognitive challenge may be used to help challenge some of the thoughts underlying TAB.

Behavioural hypothesis testing. 'Relax! Take it easy! Let someone else take the strain!' It all sounds so easy! Yet changing TAB can be a (rewarding) challenge to both patient and helper. Most people who are Type A have been this way for many years – their behaviour has typically been rewarded, perhaps financially or through career progression. Many consider their anger as being useful: 'It helps get things done'; ' I can't get people off my back without getting angry with them . . .' Thus, in encouraging people to modify their behaviour, helpers may be asking people to challenge some of their fundamental beliefs about themselves and how they have to behave. This may involve suggesting they try out a new behaviour to see whether or not it helps them to reduce their degree of stress.

For example, one office worker felt that he would be unable to work effectively if he slowed down, and only did one thing at a time. His usual practice was to switch between two or three jobs, and to have a 'busy' desk. Logically, it is possible to see that this mode of work is less effective than concentrating on one piece at a time, although he was reluctant to accept this view. Together, he and his helper negotiated a behavioural test, which allowed him to explore the value of a different way of coping with his work:

Helper: *OK. We've agreed that you find your job very tiring. You always have two or three things on the go, and are trying to juggle many different ideas in your head. I wonder if there's a way in which you could reduce some of this stress . . .*

Mr D: *I can't really see a way. I've got to keep all these things going or I won't finish my work by the end of the day . . .*

Helper: *Do you? I wonder if that's true. Have you ever tried to find out whether you have to do so many things at once? Perhaps you may be more effective if you only do one thing at a time, and keep an empty desk.*

Mr D: *I guess it's possible . . . I suppose I could try it out and see.*

Helper: *Why not try it out for a week, and see how it goes?*

He agreed for one week to keep a tidy desk and to do only one job at a time. The following week, he was able to report how his hypothesis had not been supported, and that he had been more effective and less stressed using his new approach to work, which he continued to do.

Behavioural hypothesis testing is used quite frequently in this type of intervention, as it allows people to explore new ways of coping with stressors, ways which they may otherwise have been reluctant to try.

However, only if they find the new behaviour works for them will they adopt it. This approach carries little risk, and potentially large benefits.

One particular type of behavioural change which may benefit people who engage in Type A behaviours is to deliberately engage in a more relaxed style of behaviour than they previously may have considered. This can be more proactive than simply changing responses to triggers, and incorporate planned changes, such as spending more time talking to family members, slowing down eating, or not taking work home in the evening. Such alternatives may bring about profound and sustained behavioural change. They may also reduce the number of Type A triggers to which the person is exposed, further reducing their TAB. Mr D provides an example of how behavioural changes can have beneficial social consequences.

Case Study

Although Mr D was a successful salesman, he got little intrinsic pleasure from his job. His primary motivation for going to work was to earn money. He was so busy at work that he rarely talked socially to his colleagues, and as a result of his brusqueness had lost two secretaries in the previous year.

After attending a TAB management group, Mr D began to make quite profound changes to his work habits. He began to remove the pressure of his working day by making fewer appointments each day, and moving from clear appointment times to a less time-pressured system of visiting clients 'some time in the afternoon'. This allowed more space in his day, and relieved some of the pressure and his tension. He also began to use this time to develop a more social role at work, spending more time chatting to his colleagues and secretary. Over the course of a few weeks Mr D began to enjoy his work more – and to have more help from his secretary in particular, who no longer felt harassed or resentful towards her previously over-demanding boss. This it turn reduced some of the triggers to his irritation at work, and helped to reduce his overall level of TAB.

Anger control. Anger has previously been identified as a central component of TAB. It can be seen as having at least two components: 'anger-out' which is expressed and obvious, and 'anger-in', which is anger that is held in and hidden. Anger management strategies can be useful in reducing both.

A common cause of anger is a failure to be assertive. Most of us have experienced the anger that can arise when we are given poor service in a shop, or are pushed in front of in a queue. We often say nothing at the time, and feel a mixture of anger towards the perpetrator and ourselves for not doing anything to remedy the situation. In contrast, there are situations where a relatively innocuous event results in someone totally 'losing their rag' for very little apparent reason. Both types of anger may result from a failure to be assertive. Anger-in generally results from being under-assertive, and anger-out from being over-assertive.

Assertiveness skills are an important element in anger control. If one can learn to be appropriately assertive, many anger-provoking situations can be averted or defused. Unfortunately, while these skills are relatively easy to teach (if not implement), they are beyond the scope of this book. Some useful texts are suggested in Appendix 4; Further Reading.

More pertinent to controlling the expression of anger are the skills of relaxation, guided self-dialogue, and cognitive challenge. Episodes of anger are like any other stressed response, and can be controlled using these techniques. The classic notion of anger control is to 'count to ten' – after which most people then express their anger! However, if a period of a few seconds is used to utilize stress management skills, this can make a difference. Nevertheless, because anger is such a powerful emotion, these cannot be used to maximum effect without rehearsal, and some practice in less emotionally-arousing situations.

Many anger-provoking situations arise as a result of some perceived personalized insult or inequity: 'He never does this with other people . . .'; 'Why pick on me!'; 'Every time I see him, he's rude. I'm sure he's got something against me . . .'; 'Why me?! It always happens to me, never anyone else!'. One key cognitive challenge, therefore, may be to try to rationalize these types of thoughts and think if they are *really* true, as well as using other self-dialogue and relaxation skills:

What I will do: Immediately take time to think.
Don't get hooked straight into my anger.

What I will say to myself: *'Take ten – think this through.*
Relax . . . Slow your breathing . . . don't let it take you over.
He does this to everyone . . . not just me. Don't take it personally.'

Keeping relaxed: Try to keep as relaxed as possible all over.
Remember to take deep slow breaths.
Concentrate on relaxing shoulders, arms and stomach.

Some final comments. Two final issues relating to working with people who frequently engage in TAB are worth a brief mention. Firstly, in my own work with them, I never label them 'Type A'.

Instead, we discuss such behaviour in the context of 'self-stressing' behaviours. Labelling someone as 'Type A', does not help them to identify and change their behaviour, and may make them increasingly anxious about the impact of their behaviour on their health. Second, wherever it is reasonable I try to work with Type A people in small groups, of four or five people. Such groups may be very supportive, and facilitate behavioural change more than individual counselling as group members can relate to the experiences of others as they change their behaviour, and give to and gain encouragement from them.

Summary

❏ Smoking

Four stages of giving up smoking were identified, each with a set of tactics to help the smoker pass to the next stage of stopping:

Stage 1: Thinking about giving up
Stage 2: Planning to give up
Stage 3: Starting to give up
Stage 4: Stopping
Stage 5: Long term abstinence

❏ Encouraging exercise

A number of strategies to encourage patients to maintain exercise beyond the rehabilitation gym were identified:

Programme design issues
Generalization issues

❏ Changing Type A Behaviour

Helping people to change TAB involves many of the strategies used in stress management training. Additional strategies or foci include: behavioural targeting and behavioural hypothesis testing and anger management.

6

Putting It All Together

Although this book can only introduce the reader to a number of issues and techniques in counselling, (suggested further reading is given in Appendix 4), I hope it shows the importance of appropriate communication and counselling for people both at risk for, and who have developed, heart disease.

What should also be clear is that these should be skills held by those who most frequently come into contact with patients: that is, nurses, physicians and other paramedical personnel. Appropriate emotional and psychological care cannot simply be developed by employing more counsellors to provide a specialist service. While some people would undoubtedly benefit from the expertise of such professionals, the majority of patients benefit more from appropriate care provided by those with whom they come into most contact.

Organizational Issues

Two important questions concerning the organization of counselling in health care can be identified: who should counsel, and how can organizational barriers to counselling be minimized? While some aspects of these questions have already been addressed, either explicitly or implicitly, within the previous chapters, some new issues are worth consideration, and some previously identified issues worth reiterating and drawing together.

Who should counsel – and why?

Appropriate communication is necessary by everyone involved in the care of any patient, and all should have some degree of training in such skills. A smaller number of people may be involved in counselling, but there are no strong arguments to suggest some professionals would make better counsellors than others. However, the degree and consistency of patient contact which nurses have suggests they may be the most appropriate people in most circumstances. Other professions with formal training in counselling skills, such as psychologists or social workers, may also be involved, but this should typically be only for those with particular problems.

It is important that psychological care becomes a routine aspect of patient care, and that this is monitored and co-ordinated by a designated and senior member of staff. This person may not necessarily be involved in counselling particular patients (although they often are), but will take responsibility for co-ordinating such care. In addition, they should facilitate effective communication between the different professionals involved in caring for particular patients. All those involved in the care of patients need quite high levels of information about each person, and this can only be maintained by co-ordinated inter-professional communication.

Despite an acknowledged need to improve carers' communication and counselling skills, a number of personal and organizational barriers frequently preclude the development of such skills. For example, as Fallowfield and Davis (1991) note, many specialist counsellors in medical settings are appointed on the grounds that they are kindly, well-motivated and have lots of experience with patients. While these qualities are important, they by no means guarantee that such people are necessarily good counsellors. Many carers may have experience of coping with patients but this may not have taught them adequate communication skills. In one study it was found that the agenda set by nurses focused predominantly on procedural and treatment-related topics. If nurses lacked confidence in communication, they specifically avoided talking to those who needed it the most – the distressed or dying. While this may prove adaptive in the short term (it may be inappropriate for nurses with poor communication skills to be involved with such people), it does not foster the development of appropriate skills.

A further organizational barrier to the development of appropriate communication and counselling skills may also be found higher up health care professional hierarchies; for example, it has been reported that a number of senior health professionals and managers actively resist initiatives to improve communications. This may be because 'knowledge is power': by limiting patients' knowledge about their condition and the range of possible treatments, the hegemony of the medical professions can be maintained. Patients and relatives will not challenge medical opinion (presented as fact), or engage in any decision-making about their treatment.

Time and space for counselling

It is too often true that wards, outpatient suites, and other health care settings have limited availability of facilities which allow the privacy needed for counselling. I have myself conducted counselling sessions in store rooms and even, on one occasion, a sluice. Obviously, such settings are far from ideal. The minimum provision for effective counselling should be a private room with good soundproofing and a 'Do not disturb' notice on the door. It is inappropriate to expect people to express concerns, fears, or other private issues in a public place. This includes the bedside, whether with curtains pulled around or not. It is impossible to be sufficiently private in such settings, and these should be avoided wherever possible.

Lack of time is a typical explanation for many health professionals' failure to provide adequate emotional or informational care. This reasoning is false for a number of reasons. Integrating such care into the standard treatment regime and increasing relevant professionals' skills can minimize the time that such care takes. Nevertheless, it cannot be denied that such care does take time and, if rushed, would be inadequate. A more powerful argument, is that such care is 'time-effective'. Branch (1987) found that good communication skills enhanced doctors' interest and ability to deal with patients' feelings, and by doing so helped them to talk more freely and co-operatively. This resulted in increased adherence to medical regimes and less misunderstandings and disagreements between doctor and patient. In other words, it was time well spent.

Communication and adherence

A serious problem with many treatments is that patients do not adhere to them. It may take the skills of many professionals to diagnose and treat a patient while in hospital. However, much of this is as naught if, on discharge, they fail to adhere to medical advice or take medication. Unfortunately, this is all too common. High levels of non-adherence to drug treatments – as high as 80 percent for some hypertensive medication – have been identified. While some people may stop taking drugs because of their side-effects or simply because they are forgetful, a major reason for non-adherence is poor communication.

Adherence is strongly related to the quality of communication used to give instructions and explanations. Instructions which are clear increase adherence rates. However, a number of researchers have identified that satisfaction with care in general, and communication in particular, also exerts a powerful effect on adherence. For example in one child care clinic it was found that only five percent of women rated their interactions with doctors as friendly or empathic, and only one quarter felt they were given the opportunity to discuss their main concerns about their child. This had direct implications for the care they gave their child following the consultation: 16 percent of mothers who expressed some degree of dissatisfaction with the communication with doctors adhered to the advice they were given, in contrast with 54 percent of those who were satisfied.

A further example of the benefits of appropriate communication stems from research into its impact on patients' reactions to surgery. It has been reliably found that five to ten minutes spent preparing people for what will happen to them during and following surgery can significantly reduce the amount of pain and sedative medication required in the post-operative period, and may shorten the time patients spend in hospital by as much as two or three days. A powerful effect for such a minimal intervention!

Staff support

Providing full care in acute settings, with all the potential for trauma that exists, can be extremely demanding. Although the Briggs Report of 1972 suggested that all nurses should have access to a counsellor, this has not happened. However, the lack of formal provision of counselling services should not prevent more *ad hoc* means of support being established.

The type of support need necessarily vary according to the demands made on, and strengths of, the organization in which such care is provided. Two models of support are suggested that may be implemented either separately or together. The first type can be provided through regular meetings which focus on the discussion of issues resulting from providing emotional care and counselling. These meetings may be used to talk about particular cases: key workers may seek advice, for example, on how best to handle difficult issues. They also may be used to explore different techniques and styles of communication and counselling, or simply to offer emotional sup-port to someone who has had a painful or difficult experience in counselling.

A second form of support can be gained by using a 'buddy system', whereby people may confer individually with colleagues to discuss problems they are having or to express upset, anger, or frustration at situations that have arisen during counselling. Support from a buddy need not necessarily be frequent or face-to-face. Simply knowing there is someone with whom you can talk through any issues you wish can be very supportive – even if this is by telephone.

Training issues

The need for appropriately skilled workers has a number of implications for the development and provision of health care services. Professionals need to be equipped with the means and skills to engage in appropriate emotional care, and to deal with the emotions they too may experience as a result of such care.

Although the teaching of communication and counselling skills has until recently had a low priority within the training of most health professionals, this is likely to change following recent recommendations for nurse and medical teaching made by the UK 2000 Project and General Medical Council respectively. However such training is conducted, it should incorporate a degree of supervised role-play and practice. A theoretical understanding of the principles of good communication does not ensure appropriate communication. Indeed, one study reported a *negative* relationship between medical students' understanding of the principles of good communication and their actual interview performance.

There is a need to incorporate skills teaching into the core curriculum of those involved with caring for people. There also needs to be opportunities for staff to further develop or maintain their skills following qualification. This may both increase the effectiveness of health care at the same time as minimizing the awkwardness and discomfort felt by many inadequately-trained health professionals when faced with people's distress. However, these are hopes for the future. What of the present?

In the UK health service, access to professional training in communication and counselling skills is slim. The person who wishes to develop such skills therefore has to show some initiative in finding courses, advisors, or even supervisors. Many colleges or university departments run evening or part-time courses which teach counselling and other therapy skills. Many such courses are validated by professional bodies such as the British Association for Counselling. There are also an increasing number of alternative and non-validated courses appearing, which provide an excellent level of skills training. However, a number have been criticized as being inappropriate and of little value. If in doubt, it may be worth asking other professionals such as social workers or clinical psychologists about the value of an advertised course. An alternative to long-term courses are shorter ones, which are often advertised in professional magazines (such as *The Psychologist, Nursing Times*). Again some are run by reputable bodies, such as the British Association of Behavioural Psychotherapy, and some not so reputable bodies.

There are a number of alternative, and more informal, ways of obtaining teaching and supervision in communication and counselling. One may be to contact local clinical psychology or social work departments. Some give commitment to training and supervising other professionals in counselling techniques, and it may be possible to negotiate this.

Supervision typically involves case discussions, in which actual incidents are analysed and alternative strategies thought through and discussed. While this may be of benefit to those with training and experience in counselling, this type of discussion may also be useful between staff who have an interest in communication and counselling issues, and who are prepared to present and discuss their experiences with others with a similar interest. This may not provide an expert opinion of events, but it should encourage the expression of differing opinions and approaches which would be useful to all those involved. This group may also provide emotional support should this be necessary, as well as training and expertise to members of staff with less training in counselling or communication skills.

Who should be counselled?

Almost without exception the examples of counselling examined so far have involved the patient directly. This bias may be considered rather unfortunate, because in many cases the distress and anxieties of people emotionally close to patients may be just as great, or greater, than those of the patients themselves (see Chapter 1).

Counselling couples can be a complex and skilled task, and often requires specialist training. If, for example, serious relationship problems become apparent, and the person wishes help in dealing with this, they should normally be referred to such specialists. Not only do most counsellors not have the skills necessary, but because of their closeness to one of the partners, they may have biases – such as favouring the interpretation of events by that partner – that would interfere with any counselling.

Nevertheless, it must be borne in mind that many patients' partners do have worries and concerns. The minimum provision of care should ensure that they are given opportunities to receive informational and emotional care similar to that given to the patients themselves. In some cases, problem-solving counselling or even stress management training could also be appropriate.

Referring on

Patients in both acute and preventive settings may require more psychological help than can be provided by front-line workers. Their problems may be too intractable, or their distress too great to be reduced by the brief contact usually available to such workers. Here, referral to other professionals may be needed. To minimize any delay in referral, lines of communication should be established before any crises are likely to occur. Key professional groups with whom to establish links might include clinical psychology, liaison psychiatry, and social work services. Ideally, a member of one or more of these professions should form part of a multi-disciplinary care team directly and routinely involved in care provision. A less satisfactory system would involve identified workers within one or more of these professions taking responsibility for referrals from members of the medical team.

Developing Rehabilitation Programmes

The main focus of the book has been on using techniques and strategies according to the needs and wishes of individual patients or clients. However, many patients enter rehabilitation programmes which have to meet the needs of many and various people. Such programmes inevitably involve a degree of standardization and have to be thought through carefully to be maximally effective. This section describes a patient education programme developed by Baer *et al.* (1985); a stress management based programme (Bennett *et al.*, 1991); and an innovative minimal intervention programme (Frasure-Smith and Prince, 1989).

A ward-based patient education programme

To encourage appropriate behavioural change following MI it is important that patients have a good understanding of:

- what it is appropriate and safe to do following discharge;
- how to minimize any disabilities resulting from the MI;
- how to minimize the risk of further MI.

To allow such changes to be made, some degree of patient education is inevitable. However, from a counselling perspective educational programmes must be seen as a minimal intervention: while they may help highly motivated and able people to make required behavioural changes, others may need more substantive help.

This type of programme can alert people to what should be done, and help them to make some decisions about what changes they personally wish to make. Ideally, further help should be available to enable people to make and sustain any changes, for example through attending exercise rehabilitation programmes, dietary counselling, smoking cessation, and stress management groups.

The patient education programme developed by Baer *et al.* was run in hospital before discharge. It comprised an introductory session and eight group sessions, each lasting approximately 45 minutes. The first 30 minutes of all group sessions were devoted to information giving, and the final 15 minutes were reserved for a question-and-answer period on the material presented. The format is outlined in Figure 5.

Day 1: Introduction to the course.
Day 2: Focus on physical effects of MI; cardiovascular system function.
Day 3: Physical adjustment to MI; angina and sexual function.
Day 4: Hypertension as a risk factor for MI; treatment compliance.
Day 5: Smoking as a risk factor for MI: strategies for quitting.
Day 6: Exercise, diet, and obesity as risk factors; recommendations for change.
Day 7: Stress and recovery.
Day 8: Review.

Figure 5: Format of a typical patient education programme

A typical stress management programme

Before describing some stress management programmes which have been conducted, it is important to consider the context in which these, and other, rehabilitation programmes are conducted.

Hospital-based interventions have a number of advantages – if nothing else, they give the patients something to do while in hospital! In addition, they ensure all patients can attend and reduce the problems of drop-out due to transport and other difficulties which may occur in out-patient programmes. Finally, they may provide some reassurance to patients on discharge that they have some of the skills they require to deal with some of the stresses they will face outside the hospital ward.

On the debit side, such interventions may be difficult to organize as they require high numbers of patients to ensure groups will be available to all patients while in hospital. In addition, any skills taught are necessarily learned away from the context of patients' everyday lives, and without opportunities for practice and feedback, they may prove less than maximally helpful. For this reason, it may be best to run at least some group meetings both during the in-hospital period and during the weeks immediately following discharge.

Figure 6 shows the outline of a stress management intervention we have developed.

Week 1: Introduction to the principles of stress management, including underlying physiology and model of the stress process. Deep relaxation.
Week 2: Introduction to guided self dialogue.
Week 3: Introduction to cognitive challenge.
Week 4: Review. Introduction of further relaxation and meditation techniques.
Week 5: Modifying TAB: time urgency and competitiveness.
Week 6: Modifying TAB: acute anger control.
Week 7: Assertiveness training.
Week 8: Review.

Figure 6: A typical stress management programme

Each weekly group meeting lasts approximately one-and-a-half hours, and typically involves between four and six clients. The first session begins with an introduction to the principles of stress management and an explanation of what to expect over the coming weeks. This is followed by a live deep relaxation practice. Attenders are provided with a relaxation tape, and encouraged to practise daily and keep a tension diary.

Subsequent meetings follow a similar pattern. Each begins with a discussion focusing on the successes or otherwise of attenders' attempts to use the techniques taught in the previous meeting. This is followed by fairly didactic teaching of new skills for that week, followed by discussion and role play, in which group members think about how and when these skills could be implemented, and rehearse their use.

Participants are encouraged to try out the skills during the week, and to keep a record of their progress, which they bring back to the following week's meeting to remind them of successes and failures during the discussion. If there is time, each meeting involves practice of relaxation, although this is not always possible. However, attenders are encouraged to practise deep relaxation daily for the first four weeks of the course, and an abbreviated relaxation protocol for the final four weeks. They are also encouraged to practise relaxation on an occasional basis after the group has finished. An emphasis is placed on integrating each of the various skills in effectively combating stress as the weeks progress.

A minimal intervention programme

The Life Stress Monitoring Program (Frasure-Smith and Prince, 1989) adopted a more radical approach to stress management. Its developers argued that not all patients in rehabilitation need training in stress-management techniques, nor do they necessarily need to use them at all times. Thus, they developed a minimal intervention, which was directed to patients at times of particular stress. The intervention involved monthly telephone monitoring of patients' experiences of 20 symptoms of stress, including insomnia, depressive feelings, and inability to concentrate. When a monthly call revealed five or more symptoms, or a patient was re-admitted to hospital, they received home-based interventions, conducted by nurses, to help them deal with whatever stresses were occurring at the time.

Over the year of the programme, about half the monitored patients reported sufficiently high stress levels to warrant intervention. On average, the nurse provided each high stress patient with five to six hours of contact. Interventions involved teaching about CHD and medication, counselling, providing emotional support and referring patients to cardiologists or other health professionals as required. The intervention was particularly useful for two key reasons: first, it only provided treatment on the basis of an index of need, which served both to allow resources to be placed where they were most needed and did not waste the time of patients who had no need of such help; second, it allowed each intervention to be specifically tailored to the individual needing help, which varied a great deal.

How Effective are Interventions?

The final part of the book examines the efficacy of some interventions targeted at patients in rehabilitation programmes, before briefly reviewing evidence of the effectiveness of stress management techniques in reducing hypertension, drawing on work mainly conducted in primary preventive settings.

Psychotherapy

A number of studies have compared the effectiveness of a psychotherapy and a no treatment control condition, with encouraging results. Gruen (1975), for example, reported that psychotherapy begun during the acute phase and aimed at reducing psychological distress and facilitating uptake of adaptive behaviours reduced the time spent in hospital and CCU. It also led to lower levels of anxiety and depression in comparison with controls who received no intervention.

Stress management

A number of studies have shown stress management to both ameliorate distress and enhance the rehabilitation process. For example, Burgess *et al.* (1987) evaluated an intervention targeted at three aspects of rehabilitation: limiting psychological distress (using cognitive-behavioural interventions), providing support to both patient and a key member of their social support network, and facilitating job re-entry by meetings with patients' employers or supervisors. Outcome at three- and twelve-month follow-up was assessed in comparison to patients receiving standard post-MI care. At the earlier follow-up, intervention participants reported lower mean distress scores, significantly less need for family support, and a quicker return to work than controls.

Only a few studies have attempted to identify the key therapeutic components required to bring about change. Langosch *et al.* (1982) compared the relative effectiveness of stress management training involving both cognitive and relaxation techniques, relaxation alone or a standard medical treatment condition. There was little additional advantage conferred by the cognitive procedures. Immediately following intervention, both treatment groups scored better on measures of social anxiety and speed and impatience components of TAB. Participants in the stress-management intervention reported more confidence in their ability to handle stress, while those in the relaxation condition had improved on a measure of cardiac complaints. However, by six-month follow-up there were minimal differences between the two intervention groups, although both fared better than patients who received no psychological support.

The Life Stress Monitoring Program (Frasure-Smith and Prince, 1985; 1989) was compared with a standard care intervention in 461 men recovering from MI. It was hypothesized that this stress reduction would have a direct impact on morbidity and mortality. Although there was no difference in mortality after four months, over the remaining eight months of the programme there was a 70 percent treatment-related decrease in mortality. This was achieved with just six hours' contact with high-stress patients, who in turn comprised only half of those allocated to this condition. After four years, the reductions in cardiac deaths were no longer significant, although the rate of re-infarction was significantly lower.

TAB modification

While the early work of Suinn (e.g. 1975) suggested that TAB could be modified following MI, only one study to date has investigated whether changes in TAB are accompanied by a reduction in the risk of re-infarction (Friedman *et al.*, 1986). This group compared the effectiveness of group cardiac counselling versus cardiac counselling combined with TAB modification or standard medical treatment in over 800 participants who had an infarction at least six months previously. Each group met at increasing intervals for the four-and-one-half-year life-span of the project. Cardiac counselling consisted primarily of discussions aimed at increasing adherence to prescribed dietary, exercise, and drug regimes. The TAB modification programme employed a wide variety of cognitive and behavioural techniques (including relaxation, cognitive restructuring, and behavioural assignments).

By the final assessment, the cumulative total re-infarction rate was virtually halved in the combined treatment group relative to the cardiac counselling group (12.9 percent versus 21.2 percent), and death from CHD (5.2 percent versus 7.2 percent) was also reduced significantly. Perhaps even more persuasively, participants in either group who reported significant behavioural change at the end of the first year registered a significantly lower cumulative infarction rate in the remaining three-and-one-half years in comparison with those who failed to do so (6.6 percent versus 17.2 percent). These data present powerful evidence to suggest that changing TAB will directly influence risk of re-infarction. However, it should also be noted that participants in the cardiac counselling group in turn fared better than those who received only the standard medical treatment.

Exercise training

A number of studies have examined the impact of cognitive behavioural interventions on adherence to exercise regimes. In one, 120 post-MI patients were allocated to experimental and control groups. Each group participated in a twice-weekly supervised exercise programme. Those in the experimental group took part in regular self-monitoring of variables such as weight loss, smoking habits, and activity levels using self-report diaries. By six months adherence rates in experimental and control conditions were 54 percent and 42 percent respectively.

It has been suggested that poor group leadership and a lack of group camaraderie were two key contributory factors to non-adherence. Supportive data comes from a number of studies, although for the most part these have not been conducted in the context of cardiac rehabilitation. King and Frederiksen (1984) found that encouraging subjects to jog with at least one other team member was more effective than a no treatment control condition in maintaining adherence during the course of group meetings. Another study (1984) identified both cognitive and group features as important in maintaining compliance. In a series of small studies they demonstrated that flexible goal setting and instructor support and feedback were critical in minimizing drop-out.

There is evidence that the intensity of the exercise programme may also affect the levels of stress experienced by group members and adherence. High intensity exercise has been found to increase tension, anxiety scores and drop-out. Reductions in anxiety were also reported following an exercise programme involving moderate exercise, but increased anxiety following a programme consisting of more intense exercise. However, apparently contradictory findings were reported by Norris *et al.* (1992). They found that young people who participated in high intensity exercise showed the greatest reductions in psychological stress and low drop-out rates.

Thus, the level of exercise *per se* may not be the critical factor in promoting adherence. Rather, it may be accompanying changes on psychological variables, such as mastery, associated with success in achieving or maintaining a prescribed or recommended level of exercise that is crucial. These, of course, may vary between populations. What seems to be critical is that exercise programmes are tailored to the individual abilities of participants rather than predetermined group norms.

Partner-based interventions

Despite the strong evidence to suggest that spouse involvement is a critical factor in the rehabilitation process, and that partners suffer high levels of psychological morbidity, few studies have evaluated the value of counselling. Additionally, existing research has largely been of an anecdotal nature, or of such limited scope, as to make any results difficult to generalize. One of the better studies, conducted by

Dracup (1985), compared group counselling either with patients alone, with their spouses, and a no treatment control condition. Counselling with spouses did bring about more sustained changes on measures of depression and anger, although measures of marital adjustment changed little over time. In a similar size study, Thompson and Meddis (1990) randomly assigned couples to a programme of support and counselling given on four occasions during the in-patient phase, or to routine care. Immediately following the intervention, partners in the intervention condition reported less anxiety than controls, a finding which was maintained to six month follow-up.

A further brief, but innovate procedure, was reported by Taylor *et al.* (1985). They found that wives who both saw their husband take a treadmill test and who also undertook the task themselves rated their husband's physical and cardiac capability more highly than either wives who did not see the test or who witnessed the test but did not themselves participate. Although the implications of the study were not explored by the authors, these findings suggest that participatory support may be an effective way of reassuring spouses about the capacity of their partners to safely resume customary physical activities.

Hypertension

One of the largest trials to evaluate the effectiveness of relaxation techniques in reducing hypertension was conducted by Chandra Patel and colleagues (1985). They randomly allocated over 200 volunteers to an intervention group focusing on relaxation and meditation techniques or a minimal intervention (information only) group. After eight weeks, blood pressures had fallen significantly more in the intervention compared to control group, with a mean reduction of 20 mmHg versus 8 mmHg in systolic BP and 11 mmHg versus 4 mmHg in diastolic BP. These differences were increased by three-month follow-up, and the superiority of the relaxation group continued until four-year follow-up.

A number of studies have found similar results to Patel. However, it has been argued that such results may be artifactual. Patients may have learned to relax only while their blood pressure was being measured, producing an effect only in the clinic and not generalizing to daily life. In order to examine these issues, Agras *et al.* (1983) used semi-automatic ambulatory blood pressure recorders to monitor subjects' blood pressure every 20 minutes through the working day. Immediately after treatment, differences strongly favouring the relaxation group were found for both systolic and diastolic BP both in the clinic and worksite. These differences were maintained through to one-year follow-up, suggesting that clinic measures do reflect changes in blood pressure throughout the day and that sustained reductions in blood pressure can be achieved using relaxation techniques. The effectiveness of cognitive therapy in combination with relaxation has been examined, with differences averaging five mmHg between people not receiving cognitive therapy and those taught these techniques.

There is thus strong evidence that stress management techniques may be a powerful and safe intervention, particularly in mild hypertension. They may also advantageously be used in people with moderate to severe hypertension in combination with appropriate medication.

Afterword

A number of years ago I was a student nurse studying for my SRN qualification. One incident still lingers in my mind. One day, while I was working on a radiotherapy ward, I received an invitation to come to the office of the Director of Nursing Education. Alarmed, I went to her office at the time specified. There I received a dressing down for 'unacceptable behaviour' while on placement. My 'unacceptable behaviour'? Talking too much to patients.

I hope this book has shown that talking to patients is *not* unacceptable behaviour. Indeed, it is our duty as health professionals to talk *more* to patients. This is not to encourage idle chatter, although this does have its place. Instead, we should be viewing the needs of patients not just in terms of their physical well-being but also, and equally importantly, their psychological well-being. Only by doing so will we be able to offer a comprehensive health care service and offer the possibility for many patients to achieve their maximum potential following the development of disease.

The benefits from such holistic care are not one way: the rewards and satisfaction of high quality psychological care are often as great for those who provide the care as for the patients themselves.

References

Agras, W. S., Southam, M. A. and Taylor, C. B. (1983) Long-term persistence of relaxation-induced blood pressure lowering during the working day. *Journal of Consulting and Clinical Psychology, 51,* 792–794.

Baer, P. E., Cleveland, S. E., Montero, A. C., Revel, K., Clancy, C. and Bower, R. (1985) Improving post-myocardial infarction recovery status by stress management training during hospitalization. *Journal of Cardiac Rehabilitation, 5,* 191–196.

Banks, M. (1989) Staff counselling in the National Health Service. *Counselling in Medical Settings Newsletter, 19,* 11–13.

Beevers, G. (1992) Blood pressure and heart disease. In K. Williams (Ed.) *The Community Prevention of Coronary Heart Disease.* London: HMSO.

Bennett, P. and Carroll, D. (1990) Type A behaviours and heart disease: epidemiological and experimental foundations. *Behavioural Neurology, 3,* 261–277.

Bennett, P., Wallace, L., Carroll, D. and Smith, N. (1991) Treating Type A behaviours and mild hypertension in middle-aged men. *Journal of Psychosomatic Research, 35,* 209–223.

Branch, W. T. (1987) Doctors as 'healers'; Striving to reach our potential. *Journal of General Internal Medicine, 2,* 356–359.

Burgess, A. W., Lerner, D. J., D'Agostino, R. B., Vokonas, P. S., Hartman, C. R. and Gaccione P. (1987) A randomized control trial of cardiac rehabilitation. *Social Science and Medicine, 24,* 359–370.

Cay, E. L., Vetter, N., Philip, A. E. and Dugard, P. (1972) Psychological reactions to coronary care unit. *Journal of Psychosomatic Research, 16,* 437–447.

Doll, R., Gray, R., Hafner, B. and Peto, R. (1980) Mortality in relation to smoking: 20 years' observation on female British doctors. *British Medical Journal, 287,* 967–971.

Dracup, K. (1985) A controlled trial of couples counselling in cardiac rehabilitation. *Journal of Cardiopulmonary Rehabilitation, 5,* 436–442.

Egan, G. (1990) *The Skilled Helper: Models, skills, and methods for effective helping.* Monterey: Brooks/Cole Publishing Co.

Frasure-Smith, N. and Prince, R. (1989) Long term follow-up of the Ischemic Heart Disease Life Stress Monitoring Program. *Psychosomatic Medicine, 51,* 485–513.

Fallowfield, L. and Davis, H. (1992) Organizational and Training Issues. In Davis, H. and Fallowfield, L. (Eds) *Counselling and Communication in Health Care.* London: Wiley.

Friedman, M., Thoresen, C. E., Gill, J. J., Ulmer, D., Powell, L. H., Price, V. A., Brown, B., Thompson, L., Rabin, D. D., Breall, W. S., Bourg, E., Levy, R. and Dixon, T. (1986) Alteration of type A behaviour and its effect on cardiac recurrences in postmyocardial infarction patients: summary results of the Recurrent Coronary Prevention Project. *American Heart Journal, 112,* 653–665.

Gruen, W. (1975) Effects of brief psychotherapy during the hospitalization period on the recovery process in heart attacks. *Journal of Consulting and Clinical Psychology, 43,* 232–233.

Keys, A. (1980) *Seven countries: a multivariate analysis of death of coronary heart disease.* Harvard University Press: Cambridge, Mass.

King, A. C., and Frederikson, L. W. (1984) Low-cost strategies for increasing exercise behavior: relapse prevention training and social support. *Behavior Modification, 8,* 3–21.

Langosch, W., Seer, P., Brodner, G., Kallinke, D., Kulick, B. and Heim, F. (1982) Behaviour therapy with coronary heart disease patients: results of a comparative study. *Journal of Psychosomatic Research, 26,* 475–484.

Lazarus, R. S. and Folkman, S. (1984) *Stress, Appraisal, and Coping.* New York: Springer.

Meichenbaum, D. (1985) *Stress Inoculation Training.* New York: Pergamon.

Morris, J. N., Everitt, M. G., Pollard, R. and Chave, S. P. W. (1980) Vigorous exercise in leisure time: protection against coronary heart disease. *Lancet, (ii),* 1207–1210.

Muldoon, M. F., Manuck, S. B. and Matthews, K. A. (1990) Lowering cholesterol concentrations and mortality: a quantitative review of primary prevention trials. *British Medical Journal, 301,* 309–314.

Nichols, K. A. (1984) *Psychological Care in Physical Illness.* London: Croom Helm.

Norris, R., Carroll, D. and Cochrane, R. (1992) The effects of physical activity and exercise training on psychological stress and well-being in an adolescent population. *Journal of Psychosomatic Research, 36,* 55–66.

O'Connor, G. T., Buring, J. E., Yusuf, S., Goldhaber, S. Z., Olmstead, E. M., Paffenbarger, R. S. and Hennekens, G. I. (1989) An overview of randomized trials of rehabilitation with exercise after myocardial infarction. *Circulation, 80,* 234–244

Patel, C., Marmot, M. G., Terry, D. J., Carruthers, M., Hunt, B. and Patel, M. (1985) Trial of relaxation in reducing coronary risk: four year follow-up. *British Medical Journal, 290,* 1103, 1106.

Ravnskov, O. (1992) Cholesterol lowering trials in coronary heart disease: frequency of citation and reporting. *British Medical Journal*, *305*, 15–19.

Rogers, C. R. (1957) The necessary and sufficient conditions of therapeutic personality change. *Journal of Consulting Psychology*, *21*, 95–103.

Rosenberg, L., Palmer, J. R. and Shapiro, S. (1990) Decline in the risk of myocardial infarction among women who give up smoking. *New England Journal of Medicine*, *322*, 213–217.

Roskies, E. (1988) *Stress management for the healthy Type A: theory and practice.* New York: Guilford Press.

Stern, M. J., Pascale, L. and McLoone, J. B. (1976) Psychosocial adaption following an acute myocardial infarction. *Journal of Chronic Diseases*, *29*, 523–526.

Suinn, R. M. (1975) The cardiac stress management program for type-A patients. *Cardiac Rehabilitation*, *5*, 13–15.

Taylor, C. B., Bandura, A., Ewart, C. K., Miller, N. H. and DeBusk, R. F. (1985) Exercise testing to enhance wives' confidence in their husbands' cardiac capability soon after clinically uncomplicated myocardial infarction. *American Journal of Cardiology*, *55*, 635–638.

Thompson, D. R. and Meddis, R. (1990) Wives' responses to counselling early after myocardial infarction. *Journal of Psychosomatic Research*, *34*, 249–258.

United Kingdom Central Council for Nursing, Midwifery, and Health Visiting (1992) *Code of Professional Conduct.* London: UKCC.

Appendix A: A rationale of, and preparation for, deep relaxation practice

Below are instructions that may be used to introduce relaxation methods, particularly to a group of people on a rehabilitation programme. They may, of course, be adapted to suit the particular needs of groups or individuals who are being taught relaxation methods.

'What we are going to do next is to teach you some relaxation techniques. These have proven very useful in controlling stress and helping people cope after a heart attack. Regular relaxation may also reduce the risk of having a further heart attack.

Why is relaxation so useful? One of the problems we all face in our everyday lives is dealing with stress. Some stresses, such as dealing with marital or financial problems, may be overwhelming and obvious. Other stresses (or hassles) may be less obvious. Examples of these include the hassles involved in driving to work or sitting in a crowded bus through a traffic jam, dealing with colleagues at work, coping with a crying child, and so on. Each hassle in itself is not particularly stressful. However, the overall effect of these means that by the end of the day it is easy to feel exhausted and fractious.

Coping with these hassles also affects our blood pressure and how hard our heart works. Both these functions are controlled by the nervous system. Part of the function of the nervous system is to prepare us to do something physical in response to stress; to either deal with it or, literally, to run away. This is called the flight-or-fight response. Essentially, the nervous system is built for rapid action. It has to be able to allow us to respond to emergencies, such as walking in front of a moving car, rapidly and effectively. We respond to such an event by a sudden increase in heart rate, blood pressure, and muscular tension and we (hopefully) quickly leap out of the way.

Problems occur when the nervous system responds in this way and we cannot do anything physical to either cope with or avoid the stress. For example, in a traffic jam many people become physiologically aroused and tense. You may notice that you grip the steering wheel more tightly, or show your tension in other ways. But this does not get rid of the stress. If anything, it makes it worse. Here the nervous system is still making the flight-or-fight response. If we continually respond in this way throughout the day, it is not only very tiring, it can also place a strain on the heart and contribute to the development of heart disease. Relaxation is a means of preventing this flight-or-fight response. Relaxation at times of stress dampens down this response and lowers blood pressure, reduces the strain on the heart, as well as making us feel less stressed.

The goal of teaching relaxation is that you learn to become as relaxed as possible during your daily life; in a traffic jam, during a difficult meeting with *your boss, and so on. However, to be able to do this, it is first necessary to learn to relax fully under easier conditions. This involves learning and practising deep relaxation.*

Deep relaxation consists of the systematic tensing and relaxing of muscle groups throughout the body, with the goal of becoming deeply and pleasurably relaxed. So, in a minute you will lie down (or sit in a supportive chair) and I will lead you through the exercises, telling you which muscles to tense and relax, and then allow you a few minutes of full relaxation at the end of the instructions.

As I suggested earlier, the goal of learning relaxation is to help you relax throughout the day. By this I don't mean that you have to lie down and fully relax for 20 or so minutes every time you become stressed! Rather, you should use relaxation skills to keep as relaxed as possible throughout the day; whatever you are doing.

Relaxation is a skill, just like riding a bicycle. Just like any skill, to become good requires regular practice. This involves going through the relaxation exercises, for about 20 minutes, at least once a day until you have really got the hang of them. It is important to bear in mind that if you cannot practise regularly, you will not get the full benefits of relaxation. Once you have become confident in your ability to relax under 'easy' conditions, then you can begin to relax under more difficult 'real life' conditions. However, this is for the future. Today we are going to begin to teach you deep relaxation skills.

Appendix B: Instructions for deep relaxation

The following instructions may follow on from the rationale suggested in Appendix A. They provide an approximately 20-minute routine, which is applicable to most groups or individuals in the early stages of learning relaxation. The instructions should be given in a calm, slightly soporific, voice at a steady pace with frequent pauses. This promotes relaxation and allows people to become as relaxed as possible following each instruction.

'Today I will go through the relaxation procedure with you lying down. Once you are comfortable and have loosened any tight or restrictive clothing, I will give a number of instructions. These will ask you to first tense and then relax muscle groups throughout your body. I will ask you to tense and relax each group twice before moving to the next. The muscle groups are:

- *hand and forearm – by making a fist;*
- *upper arms – by touching fingers to shoulder;*
- *shoulders and lower neck – by hunching shoulders;*
- *back of neck – by pushing back against support;*
- *lips – by pushing them together;*
- *forehead – by frowning;*
- *abdomen / chest – by holding a deep breath;*
- *abdomen – by tensing stomach muscles;*
- *thighs – by pushing together;*
- *lower leg and foot – by pointing foot up and toward head.*

Now we will begin the relaxation. First, just lie and try to relax as fully as you can for a few moments . . . Close your eyes and try to relax your whole body . . . feel it begin to get heavy and relaxed . . . Now, tense the muscles in your right forearm and hand by making a fist . . . not too tightly, but enough to feel the tension . . . study the tension . . . and relax . . . Let all the tension flow out from the muscles in your hand and forearm . . . feel the difference between tension and relaxation . . . Again, tense the muscles in your right forearm . . . hold the tension . . . and relax . . . Let the tension flow from your arm to be replaced by relaxation . . . Feel you forearm become heavy and relaxed . . . and study the difference between tension and relaxation . . . (Repeat for left forearm.)

Now tense the muscles in your right upper arm by touching your shoulder with your fingers and tensing the muscles in your upper arm . . . Hold the tension . . . and relax, resting your arm by your side . . . Feel it become heavy . . . Let go of any remaining tension, and feel the difference between tension and relaxation . . . Again, tense the muscles in your right upper arm . . . Hold the tension ... and relax, so that your upper arm becomes relaxed, comfortable and heavy ... (Repeat for left upper arm.)

Now, tense the muscles in your shoulders and lower neck by lifting your shoulders towards your ears ... Hold the tension ... and relax ... Let your shoulders and arms become as relaxed as possible ... Let the tension flow out, to be replaced by relaxation ... Feel the difference between tension and relaxation ... Once more, tense your shoulder muscles ... Hold the tension ... And relax ... your shoulders becoming as relaxed as possible ...

Now, tense the back of your neck by pushing your head gently back against the mat ... Hold the tension ... and relax ... Let the tension flow out of your neck ... Feel the difference between tension and relaxation ... Once more, tense the back of your neck ... and relax ... Let the tension flow out of the muscles to be replaced by a feeling of heaviness, warmth, and relaxation ... Feel the difference between tension and relaxation.

Now, tense the muscles in your jaw and lower face by pushing your lips together ... Hold the tension ... and relax ... Let the tension go from your jaw and lips ... Don't worry if your mouth opens a little ... This is a sign of good relaxation ... Again, tense your jaw and lips ... Hold the tension ... and relax ... Release the tension, to be replaced by relaxation.

Now, moving to the top of your head, tense the muscles here by frowning and wrinkling your brow ... Hold the tension ... and relax ... Let the tension ease away to be replaced by relaxation ... Once more, frown so that the muscles in your forehead are tense ... Hold the relaxation ... and relax ... Let all the tension flow away to be replaced by relaxation ... Enjoy that feeling of deep relaxation.

Now moving to your chest ... Tense your chest muscles by taking in a deep breath ... Hold the tension ... Note how changing your breathing feels tense and uncomfortable ... and relax ... Let your breathing become deep and relaxed and allow the relaxation to take over your whole body ... Once more hold your breath ... hold ... and relax ... Breathe deeply and easily and let the relaxation response take over, so you become more and more relaxed ... Enjoy the feeling that this brings ...

Make sure that no tension has crept into the rest of your body ... If you find any, relax it away ... so that your arms ... shoulders and neck ... and face ... are relaxed and heavy and comfortable ...

Now move your concentration to your thighs ... Tense your thighs by pushing them together ... Hold and concentrate on the tension ... and relax ... Let the tension flow away to be replaced by deep relaxation ... Once again, tense your thighs by pushing them together ... Hold the tension ... and relax ... Let all the tension flow away, so that your thighs feel warm, heavy, and relaxed ...

Now, tense your right lower leg and foot by pointing your foot up towards your head . . . Hold the tension in your foot and calf . . . Hold . . . and relax . . . Let the tension leave your lower leg to be replaced by warmth and relaxation . . . Again, tense your lower right leg . . . Concentrate on the tension . . . And relax . . . (Repeat for left leg.)

Now you have relaxed your whole body . . . Check through your body to make sure no tension has returned . . . If you find even a small amount of tension, relax it away . . . Check your arms . . . neck and shoulders . . . face . . . chest and stomach . . . thighs . . . and lower legs and feet . . . Just enjoy a few minutes deep relaxation before we draw the relaxation to an end . . .

Appendix C: An Introduction to smoking cessation

The following rationale provides explanation and some insight into strategies which may be used in a smoking cessation programme.

Giving up smoking, as you know, is not easy. However, we have identified a number of strategies that have helped many smokers to stop smoking successfully. The actual strategies that we can use differ from person to person and we will be working together to decide which are the best approaches for you. There's no point in my saying, 'Do this . . .', or, 'Do that . . .' if you don't think it will work. To help you decide whether or not to try and stop smoking with some help from me, I'll outline some of the typical things we do. But eventually, if you agree, we will work out between us exactly what you do.

Giving up smoking involves a number of stages. In the first, we try to get a good understanding of when and why you smoke. This allows us to get a better understanding of your smoking and to fine tune some of the techniques that may help. For example, this can help us to decide whether it would be useful for you to use nicotine substitutes or not. So, for the first (and easy!) week, if you agree, I suggest you don't actually try to stop smoking, but just keep a record of when and why you smoke.

After this it gets harder! You start cutting down, but only gradually. During this time you can try out a few strategies to help you cope with smoking fewer and fewer cigarettes, and we can get some idea whether nicotine substitutes would be helpful to you when you stop completely.

After a week or two of cutting down, most people find it best to stop smoking completely on one day during the following week. If you don't this tends to draw out the whole process, including any withdrawal symptoms you may experience, and it becomes increasingly difficult to stop. By then, you should have some practice in coping without cigarettes and be using nicotine substitutes if they are likely to help. Then, it's simply a matter of staying stopped!

We'll discuss each of the steps in more detail as we go along, but that's a very broad overview of what you can expect. I know it's a bit vague in parts, so if you have any questions or would like to know more about any of the aspects I've touched upon, please ask.

If asked to explain the various strategies that may be employed, the following explanation may be offered:

Everyone smokes for different reasons. However, we can identify three broad reasons. First, smokers use the nicotine in the cigarette to change their mood, to feel more alert or relaxed as they wish. Second, the need for nicotine can result in unpleasant feelings, or a craving for a cigarette, if some smokers delay too long in having one. Third, some cigarettes are smoked out of habit. You answer the phone and you have a cigarette, even though you may have smoked one a few minutes ago. All these triggers can result in a smoker having a cigarette. Some smokers, however, smoke predominantly out of habit, and some because they have a physical need for a cigarette (they are hooked).

The strategies you may use help to control the urge to smoke that results from these. Nicotine substitutes may help to reduce the craving for a cigarette. To help you cope with triggers to habit cigarettes some simple strategies such as avoiding major triggers to smoking in the few days after you stop may be helpful. Or, we can work out some simple ways of coping with triggers you can't avoid. None of the strategies is particularly sophisticated or complex. However, our experience suggests that even these simple tactics can make the difference between success and failure . . .

Appendix D: Further reading

There are a number of texts which examine in more detail some of the issues dealt with here. Some of the more useful ones include:

Risk factors and prevention
Williams, K. (Ed.) *The Community Prevention of Coronary Heart Disease.* London: HMSO.

Communication
Nichols, K. A. (1984) *Psychological Care in Physical Illness.* London: Croom Helm.

Counselling
Egan, G. (1990) *The Skilled Helper. Models, Skills, and Methods for Effective Helping.* Monterey: Brooks Cole Publishing Co.

Mearns, D. and Thorne, B. (1988) *Person-Centred Counselling in Action.* London: Sage.

Nelson-Jones, R. (1986) *Practical Counselling Skills.* New York: Holt, Rinehart & Winston.

Stress management
Dryden, W. & Golden, W. (1986) *Cognitive-Behavioural Approaches to Psychotherapy.* London: Harper & Row.

Fontana, D. (1989) *Managing Stress.* Leicester/London: British Psychological Society/Routledge.

Meichenbaum, D. (1985) *Stress Inoculation Training.* New York: Pergamon.

Roskies, E. (1987) *Stress management for the healthy Type A: theory and practice.* New York: Guilford Press.

Assertiveness training
Bower, S. A. and Bower, G. H. (1976) *Asserting Yourself: A Practical Guide for Positive Change.* Reading, MA: Addison-Wesley.

Curran, J. and Monti, P. (Eds) (1982) *Social skills training: A Practical Handbook for Assessment and Treatment.* New York: Guildford Press.

Kelly, J. A. (1982) *Social Skills Training: A Practical Guide for Interventions.* New York: Springer.

Rakos, R. F. (1991) *Assertive Behaviour. Theory, Research and Training.* London: Routledge.

General
Bennett, P. and Carroll, D. (1990) Type A behaviours and heart disease: epidemiological and experimental foundations. *Behavioural Neurology. 3,* 261–277.

Cook, D. G., Shaper, A. G., Pocock, S. J. and Kussick, S. J. (1986) Giving up smoking and the risk of heart attacks. *Lancet, (ii)*, 1345–1348.

Davis, H. and Fallowfield, L. (1992) (Eds) *Counselling and Communication in Health Care.* London: Wiley.

Frasure-Smith, N. and Prince, R. (1989) Long term follow-up of the Ischemic Heart Disease Life Stress Monitoring Program. *Psychosomatic Medicine, 51,* 485–513.

Friedman, M., Thoresen, C. E., Gill, J. J., Ulmer, D., Powell, L. H., Price V. A., Brown, B., Thompson, L., Rabin, D. D., Breall, W. S., Bourg, E., Levy, R. and Dixon, T. (1986) Alteration of type A behaviour and its effect on cardiac recurrences in postmyocardial infarction patients: summary results of the Recurrent Coronary Prevention Project. *American Heart Journal, 112,* 653–665.

Muldoon, M. F., Manuck, S. B. and Matthews, K. A. (1990) Lowering cholesterol concentrations and mortality: a quantitative review of primary prevention trials. *British Medical Journal, 301,* 309–314.

Ravnskov, O. (1992) Cholesterol lowering trials in coronary heart disease: frequency of citation and reporting. *British Medical Journal, 305,* 15–19.

Shaper, A. G., Pocock, S. J., Walker, M., Cohen, N. M., Wale, C. J. and Thomson, A. G. (1981) British Regional Heart Study: Cardiovascular risk factors in middle-aged men in 24 towns. *Journal of Epidemiology and Community Health, 39,* 197–209.

Index

adaptation, after MI 12–13
adherence to treatment 103–4
Agras, W. S. 114–15
anger 9
    control of 98–9
    see also emotions
angina pectoris 1
    and stress 56, 73–4
anxiety:
    after MI 9, 10–12
    and exercise 52, 54–5, 88–9, 114
    of partners 13, 114
    and risk factors 6–7
    see also emotions
assertiveness 98–9

Baer, P. E. 107, 108
balance sheet 49–50
Beevers, G. 2
behaviour, changing see exercise; smoking;
    stress management; Type A behaviour
behavioural hypothesis testing 97–8
Bennett, P. 5, 107
blood pressure see hypertension
brainstorming 49–50, 80
Branch, W. T. 103
Burgess, A. W. 111

Carroll, D. 5
Cay, E. L. 11
challenging 47–9, 68
    cognitive 72–4, 96
cholesterol 3
cognitive strategies for stress management
    65–74
    cognitive challenge 72–4
    and Egan counselling model 66–9
    guided self-dialogue 69–72
    and Type A behaviour 95–6
communication 16–17
    and adherence to treatment 103–4
    skills 16–17, 27–32, 102, 103
    training in 105–6
    see also counselling
confidentiality 36, 103
control, patient 31–3
coronary heart disease (CHD) 1–7
    impact of 5–14
    and psychological care 14–15
    risk factors 2–5
counselling 34–51
    and adherence to treatment 103–4
    Egan model 34–5, 36–8, 52
    helping relationship 35–6

counselling (continued)
    monitoring of 102
    for partners 106–7, 113–14
    problem-solving approach 36–50
    referring on 107
    skills and techniques 40–4, 46–50, 102
    smokers 78–80
    support for staff 104–5
    time and space for 30–1, 103
    training in 105–6
    by whom 101–2
    for whom 106–7
couples, counselling 106

Davis, H. 102
denial, of MI 8
    impact on partners 13–14
depression, after MI 9–10
    in partners 13
dialogue, self- 69–72, 99
diary:
    exercise 90
    smoking 82, 86
    tension 61–2, 64–5
    Type A behaviour 94–5
Doll, R. 3
Dracup, K. 114

education see information
effectiveness of interventions 110–15
    exercise training 112–13
    partner-based interventions 113–14
    psychotherapy 110–11
    stress management 111–12, 114–15
    TAB modification 112
Egan counselling model 34–5, 36–8, 52
    and giving up smoking 79
    and stress management 58, 66–9, 77
    and Type A behaviour 94
Egan, Gerald 34–5, 44, 52
emotions 25–33
    enhancing control 31–3
    making time 30–1
    permission to express 27–9
    safety 26–7
    sharing responses 29–30
    and stress 56
empathy 18–19, 27, 35, 42–3
exercise 4, 88–92
    and anxiety 52, 54–5, 88–9
    and boredom 90–1
    effectiveness of intervention 112–13
    and partners 114
    programme design 88–90

exercise (*continued*)
    social isolation 91
    time for 91–2
experience of MI 7–14
    partner 13–14
    patient 7–13
eye-contact 20

Fallowfield, L. 102
fear, after MI 10
fitness *see* exercise
'flight or fight' response 56
Folkman, S. 53
Frasure-Smith, N. 107, 110, 111
Frederiksen, L. W. 113
Friedman, M. 112

genuineness 35–6
goal-setting *see* problem-solving approach
Gruen, W. 15, 111
guided self-dialogue 69–72, 99

heart attack *see* myocardial infarction (MI)
heart disease *see* coronary heart disease (CHD)
helping relationship 18–20
    counselling 35–6
    and stress management 58
holistic approach 16, 115
hospitals 16–33
    communication 16–17
    emotions 25–33
    helping relationship 18–20
    information 20–5
    intervention 108–9
hypertension 2
    effectiveness of intervention 52, 114–15
    see also stress management; Type A
        behaviour

information, providing 20–5
    initial check 21–2
    information exchange 22–3
    accuracy check 23–5
    and counselling 46–7, 68
    patient education programme 107–8
interventions:
    counselling 34–51
    effectiveness of 110–15
    exercise 88–92
    hospital-based 108–9
    minimal 110
    patient education 107–8
    risk screening 5–7
    smoking 78–88
    stress management 52–77, 109–10
    Type A behaviour 92–100
    see also psychological care

Keys, A. 3
King, A. C. 113

Langosch, W. 111
Lazarus, R. S. 53
Life Stress Monitoring Program 110, 111–12

Meddis, R. 114
Meichenbaum, D. 74
minimal intervention programme 110
Morris, J. N. 4
Muldoon, M. F. 3
myocardial infarction (MI) 1
    experience of 7–14

Nichols, K. A. 21
nicotine 78–9
    substitutes 84–5, 86–7
    see also smoking
non-verbal behaviour 19–20, 29
Norris, R. 113

O'Connor, G. T. 4
organization, and psychological care 17,
    102–6

partner of patient:
    and counselling 106–7, 113–14
    effectiveness of interventions 113–14
    and exercise programmes 89, 114
    experience of MI 13–14
Patel, Chandra 114
patient:
    empowering 31–3
    experience of MI 7–13
patient education programme 107–8
posture 20
Prince, R. 107, 110, 111
privacy 36, 103
problem-solving approach 36–50
    problem exploration 37, 39–44
    goal-setting 37, 44–9
    action 37, 49–50
    and smoking 79
    and stress management 58, 66–9, 77
    and Type A behaviour 94
prompting 40–2
psychological care 17, 102
    and communication 16–17
    emotional 25–33
    helping relationship 18–20
    impact of CHD 14–15
    informational 20–5
    referring on 107
    see also interventions
psychotherapy, effectiveness of 110–11

questioning 40–2

Ravnskov, O. 3
Recurrent Coronary Prevention Project 5
referring on, for psychological care 107
reflection 76–7
reframing 67–8
rehabilitation 107–10
    minimal intervention programme 110
    patient education programme 107–8
    and stress 52, 54–5
    stress-management programme 109–10
    see also interventions
rehearsal and coping 74–6
relationship, helping 18–20
relaxation 58–65
    and daily life 62–3
    instructions 60–1, 121–3
    learning skills 59–61
    monitoring tension 61–2
    rationale for 60, 119–20
    Type A behaviour 95, 99
respect 35
risk factors in CHD 2–5
    exercise 4, 88–92, 112–13
    hypertension 2, 114–15
    screening for 5–6
    serum cholesterol 3
    smoking 3–4, 78–88
    Type A behaviour 4–5, 92–100, 112
Rogers, Carl 35
Rosenberg, L. 4
Roskies, E. 94

screening, for risk factors 5–6
self-dialogue, guided 69–72, 99
sex, after MI 12–13
skills:
    communication 16–17, 27–32, 102, 103
    counselling 40–4, 46–50, 102
    helping relationship, developing 18–20
smoking 3–4, 78–88
    counselling smokers 78–80, 124–5
    cravings 85, 87
    lapses 86
    motivation 80–1
    nicotine substitutes 84–5, 86–7
    stages of giving up 80–8

smoking (continued)
    support 84
    triggers 82–4, 86
    withdrawal effects 79, 85
staff, support for 8, 104–5
Stern, M. J. 12
stress 52–7
    model of 53–8
    and rehabilitation 52, 54–5
    responses to 53–7
    triggers 53
stress management 57–77
    cognitive challenge 72–4
    effectiveness of 111–12
    and Egan counselling model 58, 66–9, 77
    guided self-dialogue 69–72
    integrated intervention 74–7
    minimal intervention programme 110,
        111–12
    reflection 76–7
    rehearsal and coping 74–6
    relaxation 58–65
    and Type A behaviour 92–100
    typical programme 109–10
Suinn, R. M. 112
summarizing 46, 67–8

Taylor, C. B. 114
tension, physical 56
    monitoring 61–2, 64
Thompson, D. R. 114
time, for counselling 30–1, 103
training in counselling 105–6
treatment, adherence to 103–4
triggers:
    recording 61–2, 64–5, 82
    smoking 82–4, 86
    stress 53
    Type A behaviour 94–5
trust 36
Type A behaviour (TAB) 4–5, 92–100
    anger control 98–9
    behavioural hypothesis testing 97–8
    cognitive strategies 95–6
    effectiveness of intervention 112
    monitoring 94–5
    relaxation 95, 99

work, after MI 12